MIDWIFERY

JEAN L. HALLUM
BSc., M.D., D.Ch., F.R.C.O.G.
Consultant Obstetrician and Gynaecologist, Birmingham Regional Hospital Board

HODDER AND STOUGHTON
LONDON SYDNEY AUCKLAND TORONTO

ACKNOWLEDGMENTS

I am grateful to Miss S. Davy, formerly Principal Nursing Officer, Sorrento Maternity Hospital for the chapter on 'Training of Midwives'; Miss Davy has revised this chapter for the second edition. For criticism and encouragement I am indebted to friends and colleagues, particularly to the late Dr V. Mary Crosse O.B.E. The observation of patients has been of great value.

I thank Dr Danuta Gray M.R.C.O.G. for the illustrations.

Chapter 20 has been revised for the second edition by Miss M. A. Griffiths, Midwifery Divisional Nursing Officer, south area of Birmingham. For this I am most grateful.

ISBN 0 340 21124 5 Boards
ISBN 0 340 21125 3 Paperback

First Edition 1972
Second Edition 1976

Text set in 10/11 pt Monotype Bembo, printed by photolithography, and bound in Great Britain at The Pitman Press, Bath for Hodder and Stoughton Educational, a division of Hodder and Stoughton Limited, London

EDITORS' FOREWORD

The scope of this series has increased since it was first established, and it now serves a wide range of medical, nursing and ancillary professions, in line with the present trend towards the belief that all who care for patients in a clinical context have an increasing amount in common.

The texts are carefully prepared and organised so that they may be readily kept up to date as the rapid developments of medical science demand. The series already includes many popular books on various aspects of medical and nursing care, and reflects the increased emphasis on community care.

The increasing specialisation in the medical profession is fully appreciated and the books are often written by Physicians or Surgeons in conjunction with specialist nurses. For this reason, they will not only cover the syllabus of training of the General Nursing Council, but will be designed to meet the needs of those undertaking trainings controlled by the Joint Board of Clinical Studies set up in 1970.

FOREWORD

The midwife by nature of her training is capable of independent care of the woman during pregnancy and labour and of child and mother in the puerperium. In the highly sophisticated Western countries she works best as a highly skilled member of the obstetric paediatric team but in most of the world she may be the only practitioner to whom most women can turn for care.

No matter where she practises she must have a deep knowledge and understanding of the processes of human reproduction in all aspects.

Miss Hallum, who holds firm views on the quality required and status expected of the midwife, has in this excellent volume outlined the knowledge and portrayed the skills necessary for primary qualification.

Careful attention to the principles outlined and the methods and techniques portrayed will provide for the pupil a basis from which expertise can grow and on which experience can build.

PROFESSOR JAMES WALKER

CONTENTS

1 INTRODUCTION

This book has been designed as an easy-to-read textbook for midwives in training. The fact that childbirth (parturition) is a natural phenomenon is stressed. Midwives should be trained to encourage pregnant women to deliver their babies normally, the mothers remaining healthy and the babies, not just alive, but able to develop without any physical or mental handicap. *Unnecessary interference with nature can cause much harm.*

Midwives must understand the anatomy of the genital organs and the physiological changes associated with childbirth. Any abnormality must be recognised promptly, the midwife then calling medical aid, because early medical treatment can prevent many serious consequences.

Midwives have a responsible, interesting task and are allowed to conduct *normal* deliveries without direct medical supervision. As a career, midwifery has good prospects of promotion. The training is ideal for future motherhood and part-time work is available for married midwives.

Complications do arise and medical treatment is constantly changing with advancing scientific knowledge; therefore medical treatment is only dealt with briefly in this book. Routine treatment, even of the normal, changes and depends upon the consultant doctors (obstetricians and paediatricians) in maternity hospitals. Midwives should be encouraged to think and produce helpful suggestions for the Consultant doctors to consider. Joint discussion between midwives and doctors is essential to achieve the optimal care for patients.

Equipment is not detailed, because nowadays pre-packed sterilisation is done in central units. Midwives must be familiar with all apparatus required for normal and emergency therapy.

2   THE TRAINING OF MIDWIVES

The history of midwifery and the activities of the midwives of the past make fascinating and often salutary reading. Their origin belongs somewhat obscurely to the realms of pre-history. Midwives are referred to and even mentioned by name in the Old Testament and midwives of ancient Greece and Rome, in common with medical practice of the times, show some degree of enlightenment and respect for cleanliness.

The barbarous practices of the dark ages continued in England long after the Renaissance had introduced a degree of culture and only very gradually was any sort of formal midwifery training instituted. From the 16th century onwards a few unsuccessful attempts were made to introduce organised training or state recognition, but almost all the important advances have come in the last hundred years.

In 1867 Florence Nightingale brought her reforming zeal to bear upon midwifery and it was unfortunate that a school of midwifery which she established at Kings College Hospital had to be closed when a serious outbreak of puerperal infection occurred.

Largely through the writings of Dickens the public was made increasingly aware of the deplorable conditions of poverty and squalor of home confinements and the ignorance and incompetence of many of the midwives of the time. By 1872 the Obstetrical Society of London had organised a midwifery training and was conducting an examination and granting to successful candidates certificates of competence to attend normal confinements. Strenuous efforts were being made to obtain state recognition and registration for midwives. In 1881 the Midwives Institute was set up to secure better education and status. Between 1890 and 1900 eight Midwives Bills were introduced into the House of Commons but all were turned down.

The Central Midwives Board

A ninth Bill, in 1902, was passed and became the Midwives Act under which the Central Midwives Board was set up and its responsibilities defined: namely to frame rules, to regularise the training and practice of midwives, to conduct examinations and to maintain a roll of women certified as midwives. Since its inception the Board has thus exercised overall supervision of the training of midwives and of their practice. It is notable that state registration of nurses was not to come until 1919.

The training is designed to equip the student to take responsibility for the normal patient during pregnancy, labour and the puerperium and to care for the normal baby. Clearly she must understand any departure from the normal pattern, since in this event she must consult a doctor; at the same time she must be prepared to cope with any emergency arising in the doctor's absence. The line separating normal from abnormal, once sharply defined, is nowadays much less clearly distinguishable; and in practice, while the roles of doctor and midwife are mutually complementary, there are necessarily overlapping areas. In recent years the midwife's responsibilities in the field of education have received increasing emphasis and the scope of her work continues to widen as knowledge advances. The Central Midwives Board has recently defined the role of the midwife as follows:

A midwife is a person who is qualified to practise midwifery. She is trained to give the necessary care and advice to women during pregnancy, labour and the postnatal period. She is also trained to conduct normal deliveries on her own responsibility and to care for the newly born infant up to 28 days of life.

At all times she must be able to recognise the warning signs of abnormal and potentially abnormal conditions which necessitate referral to a doctor, and to carry out emergency measures in the absence of medical help.

Her work also includes family planning and certain aspects of gynaecology, in particular the conditions relating to early pregnancy. The midwife's sphere of practice may take her into hospitals, health centres, clinics, surgeries and the patient's home. In any one of these situations she has an important contribution to make in the field of health education, allaying fears and problems, counselling, giving advice and teaching on many topics relating to parenthood.

Advances in knowledge and changing social conditions have necessitated many modifications in the training and practice of midwifery. Further Midwives Acts have been passed in 1918, 1926 and 1936, while in 1951 a consolidating Midwives Act was passed, repealing all previous legislation.

Midwifery training, conducted in approved training schools, is mainly in a maternity hospital or unit, but includes 12 weeks community experience. The Board appoints educational supervisors, who visit and report on training schools, initially before approval is granted and subsequently at two-yearly intervals. The Board also conducts examinations and appoints a panel of obstetrician and midwife examiners for this purpose.

The Central Midwives Board consists of 17 members, appointed by various interested bodies for their knowledge of the training and practice of midwifery. The Department of Health and Social Security appoints seven members, three of whom are midwives, while one is a general practitioner; the Royal College of Midwives appoints four of its members; the Royal College of Physicians, the Royal College of Surgeons, the Royal College of Obstetricians and Gynaecologists and the Faculty of Community Medicine one member each; and two members, not midwives, are appointed by the National Association of Hospital Administrators in England and Wales and the Society of Community Medicine respectively. The present chairman is a midwife.

The Board's offices in Harrington Gardens, Kensington, are in Iolanthe House, a fine Victorian mansion, once the property of W. S. Gilbert, the librettist. Though the constitution of the Board has altered little, the scope of its work has increased tremendously over the years.

Practising midwives are required by the Board's rules to undertake a 'refresher' course every 5 years; these courses, organised mainly by the Royal College of Midwives, must have the Board's approval. A Midwife Teachers Diploma was introduced in 1936 and for this courses are approved and examinations are conducted by the Board. Midwifery training schools in various Commonwealth countries are seeking the Board's approval for their training and this necessitates carefully planned visits by the Board's educational supervisors. An Advanced Diploma in Midwifery conducted by Sorrento Maternity Hospital for some years under the auspices of the Royal College of Midwives and the Birmingham Regional Hospital Board received in 1971 the seal of approval of the Central Midwives Board and courses for this diploma are now more widespread.

Midwifery Training and the Student Midwife

The midwifery training which was statutorily introduced in 1902 lasted only three months. Since then its scope and depth have gradually expanded, so that in 1926 there was an increase to 6 months and in 1936 to 12 months for state registered nurses. State enrolled nurses and direct entry students, i.e., non-nurses, receive appropriately longer trainings.

Training under the 1936 Midwives Act was divided into two parts: a 6 months first period of training, a good introduction for those nurses who wanted an insight into midwifery, but who did not propose to practise; and a six months second period, giving wider experience and a chance to gain self-confidence for those who did. State enrolled nurses and direct entry students would receive respectively a 12 and 18 months first period of training; all would be at about the same level to join together for the 6 months second period of training, for which, at the time, generous domiciliary experience was available. This training, introduced at the end of 1938, survived remarkably well the hazards of World War II, with which it was soon to be beset.

In 1961, after discussions together, the General Nursing Council and the Central Midwives Board introduced jointly a plan for obstetric nurse training, to provide a short period of midwifery experience for student nurses, at approved midwifery training schools. This 3 months training, implemented by the Central Midwives Board, would provide sufficient knowledge and experience of midwifery for those nurses who did not wish to practise, but who needed some acquaintance with the subject. At the same time, it would pave the way for the introduction of a single period of midwifery training and the gradual phasing out of the two separate periods.

It was in 1968 that a single period training was introduced, at first experimentally, and then, after a successful trial period, more extensively. Most training schools have now changed over to the single period of training. While the first period of training, which had proved somewhat expensive of time, money and experience is now virtually over, the second period is expected to continue a little longer.

The present single period training for state registered nurses and registered sick children's nurses is completed within 12 months, including 5 weeks annual leave and the qualifying examination.

The first 16 weeks are spent in hospital. After a short introductory period the student concentrates on learning the pattern of normal midwifery, in theory and practice. Inevitably she will encounter a few complications. This serves merely to underline the fact that the training exists to benefit the patient and the patient can hardly be expected to fit precisely into a plan of training.

The next part of the training is the 12 weeks community assignment, during which the student is able to broaden her concept of the normal reproductive cycle, seeing it against the background of a programme of community care, with planned lectures, talks and visits dealing with the social aspects of midwifery and related subjects.

The final 19 weeks of training are again in hospital. The student midwife now consolidates her existing knowledge, takes more responsibility for her patients and gains self-confidence, at the same time learning more of the complications to mother and baby.

The qualifying examinations come at present during the 47th and 50th weeks of training. This means that the whole of the training syllabus, any house examination or final assessment and 3 weeks holiday should all be completed before the 47th week. The 51st and 52nd weeks are taken as annual leave and, with this exacting programme, it is understandable that the Central Midwives Board should require that the Halsbury award of an extra 9 days holiday be taken after the end of the 52nd week.

Even so, training schools are experiencing increasing difficulty in squeezing an ever widening programme into a steadily diminishing period of time. For this reason alone, there is a strong case for increasing the duration of midwifery training, perhaps by 3 months. A further argument in favour of longer training is the need to come to an appropriate agreement with other European Economic Community countries, in order to achieve a satisfactory pattern of reciprocity. Finally, the implementation of the Brigg's Committee's recommendations will create a need for some modifications in training patterns.

For state enrolled nurses, midwifery training lasts 18 months. The first 6 months are spent covering an introductory programme resembling obstetric nurse training but permitting further detail and wider practical experience. Direct entry students undertake a 12 months preliminary course which includes an 8 weeks introduction to basic nursing, an obstetric nurse training syllabus, a 13 weeks secondment in a general nurse training school, with experience in paediatric and female medical, surgical and gynaecological wards with appropriate theoretical instruction; and a final period of further experience of practical midwifery.

At the end of this preparatory period of 6 months, the state enrolled nurse, or one of equivalent grade is prepared for full participation in the standard 12 months course for the basic midwifery diploma. The direct entry student is similarly qualified at the end of the 12 months preparatory period.

A second type of obstetric nurse training has been recently introduced in order to meet a particular demand. This is an alternative course lasting 8 weeks and designed for male or female student nurses. Hospitals approved for obstetric nurse training may undertake either the 12 week course or the 8 week course, but not both simultaneously.

In Scotland midwifery training and practice is governed by the Central Midwives Board for Scotland, while in Northern Ireland the Northern Ireland Council for Nurses and Midwives controls both nursing and midwifery. In both of these countries midwifery training follows a pattern very similar to that in England. With much smaller populations there are, of course, fewer training schools. Thus, in both Scotland and Northern Ireland the change-over from first and second period training to the twelve months single period training could be effected quickly and has now been established for some years.

Midwifery Practice

Of the 86 000 midwives whose names are on the Central Midwives Board's Roll, almost 21 000 are practising in England and Wales and many in other countries. Of the midwives—nearly 4000—who become qualified each year, about 53 per cent practise in this country for a year or more.

The gaining of a midwifery qualification opens up a wide choice of careers, particularly to the woman who is also a state registered nurse. Whether in hospital or in the community, the midwife works within the framework of a large and sometimes complex team of specialists: in the community, general practitioner obstetricians, health visitors, community nurses and many others, including a wide variety of social workers; in hospital, not only does the midwife work with obstetricians, paediatricians, physiotherapists, social workers, radiographers and anaesthetists, but with pathologists and biochemists. The many community midwives who bring their patients into hospital for delivery make these additional contacts, while the introduction for them of duty rotas and shifts has done much to ease the strain of long hours on call.

It may be only with increasing experience that a midwife is able to decide upon the particular type of career she wishes to follow. Broadly there are three possibilities for a competent person: administration, in which, ideally, practical experience in hospital and community is coupled with advancing management courses, leading to the post of Divisional Nursing Officer, District Nursing Officer, even Area Nursing Officer and, for the extremely able midwife administrator, perhaps Regional Nursing Officer; teaching, for which, after a fairly short period of practical experience, the midwife undertakes one of a number of slightly differing courses leading to a Midwife Teachers Diploma qualification, increasingly responsible posts as Midwifery Tutor; a first-class tutor may become Director of an educational department, an Educational Supervisor to the Central Midwives Board, or a tutor in a College of Further Education, while for a graduate, a university appointment is possible; for the midwife who prefers the clinical field of work, the Advanced Diploma in Midwifery provides a stepping-stone (sometimes as an alternative to the Midwife Teachers Diploma), to a senior post in a labour ward or special care baby unit. The Central Midwives Board is emphasising the need for midwives to acquire special skills in the clinical field and it is now accepted that intravenous injections, episiotomy, with, in appropriate circumstances the subsequent repair, endotracheal intubation of the apnoeic neonate and 'topping-up' of epidural analgesia may be included in the midwife's responsibilities. Courses in special and intensive baby care, family planning, intensive therapy and other specialties provide good instruction and experience.

At present, it is relatively easy for a midwife to move from the area of teaching to that of administration, though, if the Briggs Committee's recommendations are implemented on the lines proposed, these areas will function separately, so that the lines of advancement will be more sharply defined.

Many opportunities for foreign travel are available to midwives, whether with scholarships or bursaries for study abroad, or by obtaining posts in other countries.

Many midwives go abroad immediately after qualifying. Indeed, some, often experienced nurses, undertake midwifery training with this in mind: to command a higher post in a Commonwealth or foreign country or to take on missionary work. Others, immigrants from developing countries, return home in order to work to raise the standard of midwifery practice. Many stay to study for the Midwife Teachers Diploma after which they may return to set up training schools.

Up to the present, comparatively little interchange has occurred between the United Kingdom and the other European Economic Community countries, largely on account of the many differing trainings and the consequent difficulty in securing a suitable pattern of reciprocity. This important problem is soon to be the subject of full discussion and, it may be envisaged, in due course, the enactment of legislation which should greatly facilitate these exchanges.

Professional Bodies

Of the various professional organisations and trades unions to which midwives may belong, the Royal College of Midwives is the only one which is solely concerned with the interests of midwives. It was founded in 1881 as the Midwives Institute for the purpose of improving education and practice in midwifery. In 1941 the Midwives Institute became the College of Midwives and in 1947 the Royal College of Midwives. The aim of the College, from its earliest days, has been to improve the midwifery service to the mother and baby and, to effect this, to further the education of the midwife.

The Midwife Teachers Diploma began in an informal way with a series of lectures given at the Midwives Institute in 1918. These lectures proved very popular and were continued year by year, gradually expanding, until in 1923 the Institute Teachers Committee was giving serious consideration to the question of a formal qualification for teachers. In 1925 the Midwives Institute made a recommendation to this effect to the Central Midwives Board and, the following year, organised the first examination for Midwife Teachers. Twenty-nine per cent of the candidates were successful and were awarded a Diploma. This continued until, in 1936, the Central Midwives Board set the course on a statutory basis, and took over the examination.

More recently, in 1966, a course in advanced clinical midwifery, with appropriate teaching, was introduced at Sorrento Maternity Hospital, sponsored by the Birmingham Regional Hospital Board and by the Royal College of Midwives. This continued year by year and, at the end of the 1971 course, observers from the Central Midwives Board attended the terminal examination. The successful candidates were recognised by the Board and were awarded the Board's Advanced Diploma in Midwifery. Under the Board's auspices, this course has continued in London and Birmingham and has extended to a number of other provincial towns.

As well as being concerned with Management Courses, Family Planning Appreciation Courses and other formal education, the College offers a great deal of education and counselling on an informal basis, assisting members in everything from supposedly unfair dismissals to overseas assignments.

Finally, one of the College's most important functions is to represent the midwife on the Nurses and Midwives Whitley Council, which deals with the salaries, status and conditions of service of all professional people, other than doctors, working in the Health Service.

The Salmon Committee's recommendations, revolutionary at the time of their introduction in 1966, are now fully accepted as a logical and comprehensive plan for progress through the senior grades of nursing and midwifery. The reorganised National Health Service was introduced in 1974 and is seen to be taking shape. This massive reconstruction was bound to encounter problems, financial and otherwise, during its implementation. The result is to be shown in good patient care in all areas, including that of midwifery. The Halsbury award, made in 1974, has for the first time given nurses and midwives really good salaries and conditions of service. Meanwhile, the implementation of the Briggs Committee's recommendations is awaited; and an easier and less restricted exchange and transfer of United Kingdom midwives among the other European Economic Community countries is to be anticipated with interest.

3 FEMALE GENITAL ORGANS

EXTERNAL GENITALIA (VULVA)

These are distinctive from 12 weeks fetal development, and by term it is normally easy to tell a mother the sex of her newborn baby.

Shortly before the menarche (when menstrual periods begin) there is further growth of the labia and hair appears at the mons pubis, the hair line ending horizontally on the lower abdomen. In the male, abdominal hair is triangular in distribution, the apex rising towards the umbilicus.

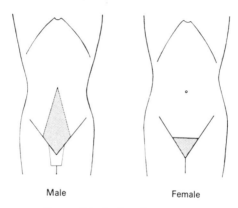

Male   Female

FIG. 3.1 Distribution of pubic hair

The Labia

The outer labia majora (right and left labium) are covered with skin, containing fat, hair and sebaceous glands. The labia unite anteriorly above the clitoris or rudimentary penis, a sensitive area, and posteriorly at the perineum. The posterior third of each labium contains a Bartholin's gland which secretes mucus to lubricate the vulva. On parting the labia majora, smaller folds of mucous membrane (*labia minora*) are seen. These are devoid of hair. Anteriorly they surround the clitoris and posteriorly unite at the posterior fourchette, the posterior entrance to the vagina.

THE VAGINA

This is the passage leading from the vulva to the uterine cervix. In a virgin the entrance (or introitus) may be partially covered by the hymen, a fold of mucous membrane. The hymen may rupture on intercourse when bleeding can occur, or occasionally the hymen has to be incised or stretched to permit intercourse. The vagina is lined by smooth squamous epithelium arranged in folds (rugae) to allow stretching during labour. The posterior wall is longer (10 cm) than the anterior

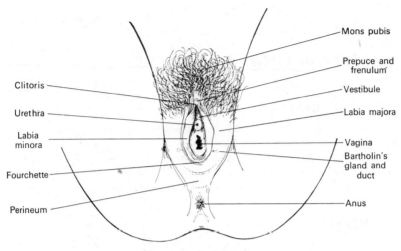

FIG. 3.2 External genitalia

(7·5 cm). Usually these walls are in close apposition. The upper end of the vagina (the vault) is divided by the cervix into four fornices, two lateral, an anterior and a posterior. The vaginal epithelium does not contain any glands, but the vagina is lubricated by cervical mucus. This secretion is acid, due to the production of lactic acid by Döderlein bacilli, which are normal residents in the vagina. The type of vaginal epithelial cell varies with oestrogen and progesterone activity.

Relations of the Vagina

These are important:
(1) *Anterior.* The upper third lies behind the bladder base and the lower two-thirds behind the urethra.

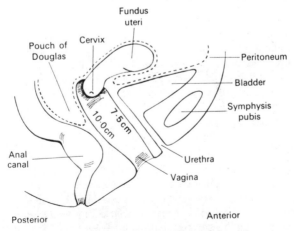

FIG. 3.3 Anterior and posterior relations of the vagina

(2) *Posterior*. The upper third lies in front of the Pouch of Douglas, the middle third in front of the rectum, and the lower third in front of the anus.

(3) *Lateral*. At the vault the ureters are in close proximity to the vagina. Lower lie the pelvic floor muscles ending on the perineum.

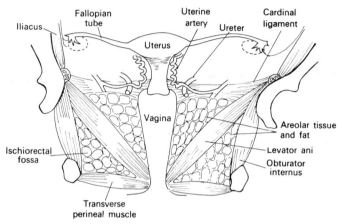

FIG. 3.4 Lateral relations of the vagina

In the connective tissue surrounding the vagina, rudimentary male reproductive organs occasionally occur and rarely produce cysts. (Gäertner and Skene)

THE PELVIC FLOOR MUSCLES

Because a human stands upright, nature has designed a support for the abdominal contents. This is provided by the pelvic floor muscles 'levator ani' which arise from the 'white line' near the ischial spines of the pelvis. These muscles are attached posteriorly to the sacrum and coccyx, and anteriorly to the symphysis pubis joining in the median line making a solid layer with a gutter shape if looked at from above.

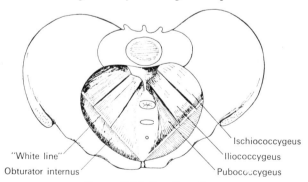

FIG. 3.5 Pelvic floor from above

The shape is important during labour. The muscles end on the perineum. The pelvic floor is perforated anteriorly by the urethra, centrally by the vagina and posteriorly by the rectum. The pelvic floor must be able to stretch during labour.

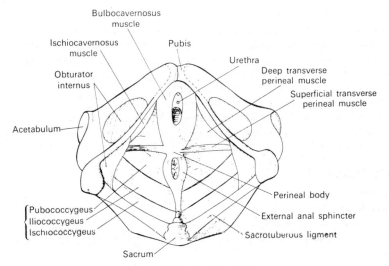

FIG. 3.6 Pelvic floor from below

THE UTERUS

This develops in two halves and these usually unite early in foetal life; occasionally a septum persists. The uterus is a pelvic pear-shaped organ and is anteverted and anteflexed, this position being maintained by ligaments. The most important are the transverse cervical (cardinal) ligaments, which pass from the cervix to the lateral pelvic wall fascia. The round ligaments arise near the uterine cornua and pass anteriorly and laterally to the inguinal canals. Posteriorly there are two utero-sacral ligaments.

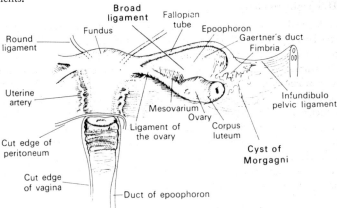

FIG. 3.7 Uterus and appendages from behind

A non pregnant uterus weighs about 510 g. Its length approximates 7·5 cm, width (between the uterine cornua) 5 cm and depth about 2·5 cm. The uterus is divided into the fundus—above the insertion of the Fallopian tubes at the cornua—

the body, and the cervix which protrudes into the vagina. The uterus is a muscular organ, but only in pregnancy are three distinct muscle layers apparent. The outer longitudinal involuntary muscles pass from each uterine cornu up to the fundus and down to near the cervix where the peritoneum is loosely attached to the anterior uterine wall. The muscles should act in unison. Deeper in the uterine wall figure-of-eight involuntary muscles enclose uterine arteries and veins. Voluntary muscles are present around each uterine cornu and just above the internal cervical os. The uterine lining or endometrium changes throughout the menstrual cycle under the influence of ovarian hormones. In pregnancy the endometrium is termed decidua and represents the result of excessive progesterone activity.

THE CERVIX

This is the lower portion of the uterus and projects into the vagina, pointing down and backwards. In the vagina, the cervix is covered by smooth squamous epithelium. The cervical canal, between the external and internal os, is lined by columnar epithelium. The cervical glands secrete mucus and during pregnancy are extremely active.

THE FALLOPIAN TUBES

These arise at the uterine cornua and pass laterally between folds of the broad ligaments to end in the peritoneal cavity as fimbria and there a ligament attaches each to the ovary. The uterine portion of the tube is termed interstitial, the middle third the isthmus and the outer the fimbria. The Fallopian tubes are lined by ciliated epithelium which helps to waft the ovum towards the uterine cavity. The fimbria resembles a sea anemone and sucks the ovum into the tube after the ovum has left the ovary. Each tube is approximately 10 cm in length with a narrow lumen.

OVARIES (right and left)

These develop in the abdomen and descend early in fetal life to the pelvis, occupying fossae in the lateral pelvic walls. The ovaries receive blood from the ovarian arteries which are branches of the aorta. The ovaries lie posterior to the broad ligaments but near to the fimbrial ends of the Fallopian tubes. The ovaries are almond-shaped, about 2·5 cm in length, and consist of an outer cortex and inner medulla. The cortex, in a young baby, contains numerous primordial follicles but these remain quiescent until the menarche. The deeper ovarian medulla consists of fibrous tissue but is haemorrhagic containing blood vessels, nerves and lymphatics. The ovarian arteries communicate with the uterine arteries. The left ovarian vein enters the left renal vein and the right the inferior vena cava. The ovaries are not covered by peritoneum, lying inside the peritoneal cavity. The infundibulo-pelvic ligaments attach each ovary to the lateral pelvic wall.

THE PERITONEUM

This is a smooth membrane lining the abdominal cavity and enveloping organs there, mainly intestines, so that they move freely without friction. The peritoneum passes from the anterior abdominal wall to cover the bladder and continues to the anterior surface of the lower part of the uterus above the cervix. The peritoneum is closely adherent to the upper anterior surface of the uterus and covers the fundus and the posterior surface, descending to the Pouch of Douglas close to the rectum and posterior vaginal fornix.

Laterally the peritoneum (anterior and posterior folds) passes to the lateral walls of the pelvis and the folds are termed 'the broad ligaments'. The peritoneal covering of the uterus has been graphically described as a sheet covering a man with outstretched arms and wiggling fingers. The man represents the uterus, the arms the Fallopian tubes, the fingers the fimbriae which leave the broad ligament and enter the peritoneal cavity.

Within the broad ligaments the uterus receives nutrition from the uterine arteries. They enter laterally above the cervix and pass upwards sending off branches which enter the uterine substance. Before reaching the uterus each uterine artery passes in front of a ureter. Uterine veins return blood from the uterus and lie close to the uterine arteries. Lymphatics also lie close to the uterine blood vessels and pass to the internal iliac glands.

THE PERINEUM

This is a triangular area between the posterior fourchette and the anus. The perineum is covered by skin, below which are the superficial perineal muscles and deeper levator ani. Around the anus the deep muscles form the sphincter ani. The perineum is sensitive, the nerve supply coming mainly from the pudendal nerves. The perineum has to stretch during labour to allow the fetus to be born. Pressure on the perineum by the fetus makes the mother desire to bear down. The perineum may tear at delivery but care at the time of delivery can prevent this.

Perineal tears are described as degrees:

    1st degree —Perineal skin torn.
    2nd degree —Perineal skin and muscles torn.
    3rd degree —Anal sphincter or anal mucosa torn.

URINARY TRACT

Because this is so close to the genital tract midwives must understand the urinary system.

The Kidneys (right and left)

These excrete waste products including water. Both are situated laterally behind the peritoneum in the upper abdomen, the right slightly lower than the left. Each kidney is enclosed by a fibrous capsule and has a typical shape. Above each kidney lies a suprarenal gland. Each kidney consists of a cortex, medulla and pelvis. From the pelvis the ureter emerges, passing down to the bladder. In order to function the kidneys require a good blood supply. This comes from the renal arteries, branches of the aorta, the renal arteries entering the renal medulla. The renal cortex is highly complex, consisting of glomeruli and tubules (loops of Henle). In every person the blood chemistry should remain constant. When the blood contains a chemical (electrolyte) greater than normal this will be filtered through the kidneys and excreted in the urine, e.g. if the blood glucose level exceeds 160 mg per cent (42 S.I. units), glucose is excreted in the urine. Some water is reabsorbed by the kidney tubules and passes back into the blood.

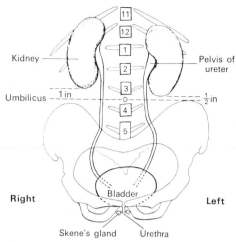

FIG. 3.8 The urinary tract in relation to the skeleton

The Ureters

These pass from each kidney pelvis down to the bladder trigone. In passage the ureters cross the pelvic brim and come close to the uterine arteries. During pregnancy the ureters dilate under the influence of the hormone relaxin; the right ureter is liable to be compressed by the growing uterus, the left is more protected because the pelvic colon lies between this ureter and the pelvic brim. If a ureter becomes compressed, the flow of urine from above diminishes and infection is liable to occur.

The Bladder

This is a muscular organ, capable of distension, storing urine received from the ureters; the outflow of urine is under neuro-muscular control. Urine is voided through the urethra. Normally the bladder is a pelvic organ but when distended rises into the abdomen. This occurs during labour. The bladder is wedge-shaped and the base is termed 'the trigone'. From the apex of this the urethra leaves and passes to the vulva.

The amount of urine excreted depends upon the patient's fluid intake. In cold weather more urine is passed, because less fluid is lost through the skin by perspiration.

Normally urine is a clear, straw-coloured fluid. It is usually acid (pink to litmus paper) but may be alkaline (turning litmus paper blue). Sometimes an acid urine appears cloudy because of urates, but this clears on boiling. An alkaline urine can be cloudy because of phosphates; these disappear on adding a few drops of 5 per cent acetic acid. Urine contains urea, sodium and chlorides. Normal urine contains no protein, glucose or acetone. The specific gravity is normally between 1·010 and 1·025.

THE FEMALE PELVIS

Before birth the fetus has to pass through the maternal bony pelvis. This will be described in some detail. The pelvis consists of three main parts:

(1) Innominate—comprising 2 iliac bones, 2 ischial and the pubis, all fused together.
(2) The sacrum.
(3) The coccyx.

Anteriorly the pubic bones are joined by a ligament, the symphysis pubis. This is about 3·7 cm long. From the upper border the pubic ramus passes laterally and backwards, uniting with the ilium at the ilio-pectineal eminence. At the lower end of the symphysis pubis, each pubic bone arches down and laterally, to fuse with the ischium. The arch ends below at the ischial tuberosities, the solid bone which supports the pelvis in the sitting position. The ischial tuberosities are usually about 11 cm apart, giving a subpubic angle of 90 degrees. The ischium joins the ilium and pubis forming part of the acetabulum of the hip joint. From the inner surface of each ischium a bony spine projects. These spines are more prominent in the male. From the ischial spine the sacrosciatic notch (an upward curve) passes to the sacrum. The wider this notch, the longer is the antero-posterior depth of the pelvis.

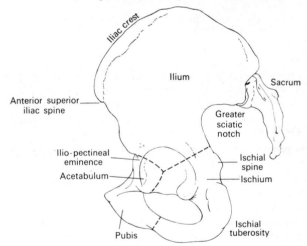

FIG. 3.9 Lateral aspect of the pelvic girdle (innominate bone)

The Ilium

Two bones form a large upper portion of the pelvis, the inner surface being smooth and concave forming the iliac fossae. The upper bony ridge or crest can be felt through the skin. This crest ends at the anterior superior iliac spines and at the posterior iliac spines, palpable as a skin dimple. The lower part of the ilium joins the ileo-pectineal line and more posteriorly the sacrum at the sacro-iliac joints.

The Sacrum

This begins at the sacral promontory and curves backwards before ending at the sacro-coccygeal joint. The sacrum consists of five fused vertebrae. Lateral to the vertebrae there are four openings (foraminae) through which sacral nerves emerge. The backward sacral curve means that on an internal pelvic examination the sacrum feels concave and smooth. Lateral to the sacral vertebrae the sacral alae unite with the iliac bones at the sacro-iliac joints.

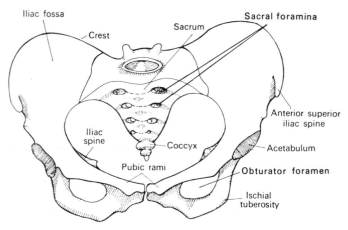

FIG. 3.10 Antero-posterior view of pelvic girdle

The Coccyx

The coccyx (rudimentary tail) is partially mobile and therefore should not interfere with labour.

Planes of the Pelvis

Laterally the pelvis is partially devoid of bone. The obturator foramen lies between the pubis and ischium. Through this opening the obturator nerve passes. Further back there are two ligaments, the sacro-iliac and the sacro-tuberous. Through the upper opening, vessels and nerves pass to the lower limbs. Through the lower opening, the pudendal nerve curves round the ischial spine to supply the perineum. From an obstetric point of view, the upper ilium (false pelvis) causes no difficulty. The first obstruction occurs at the *pelvic brim (inlet)*. This is described as a plane passing from the upper posterior border of the symphysis pubis, along the ileo-pectineal line to the sacro-iliac joint, thence to the sacral promontory posteriorly. Each side should be symmetrical.

Average measurements of the pelvic brim are as follows:

Antero-posterior. Upper border of symphysis pubis to the sacral promentory, 11 cm.
Oblique. Right and left. From one sacro-iliac joint to the opposite ileo-pectineal line, 12 cm.
Transverse. The widest distance between the ileo-pectineal lines, about 13 cm. This tranverse diameter is nearer to the sacrum than to the symphysis pubis. In the upright position the sacral promentory lies about 9·5 cm above the symphysis pubis. At the pelvic brim the fetus passes downwards and backwards.

A *mid pelvic plane* is described. This arises from the middle of the symphysis pubis anteriorly passing laterally to the ischial spines and to the junction of the 2nd and 3rd sacral vertebrae posteriorly. The shape is approximately circular, both antero-posterior and transverse diameters averaging 12·0 cm. At this level the fetus passes directly downwards.

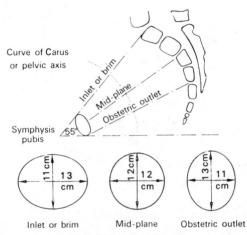

Curve of Carus
or pelvic axis

Symphysis
pubis

Inlet or brim   Mid-plane   Obstetric outlet

FIG. 3.11 Planes of the pelvis

The fetus leaves the pelvis at the *outlet*. This plane is from the lower end of the symphysis pubis to the ischial tuberosities and thence to the last sacral vertebra. At the outlet the fetus moves forwards as well as down. The widest diameter at the outlet is the antero-posterior, from the lower border of the symphysis pubis to the last sacral vertebra and averages 13 cm in length. The transverse diameter between the ischial tuberosities averages 11 cm. The passage which the fetus follows through the pelvis is known as the 'curve of Carus'.

BREASTS

At an early stage of fetal development the linea lacta forms from the axilla to the groin, and this explains the occasional presence of an axillary mammary tail in the adult. It also explains occasional accessory nipples in this line.

After about 5 months, in the fetus, epithelial cells from the skin invert, producing a rudimentary nipple which connects by ducts to rudimentary glands. By 7 months, the ducts branch to produce primitive lobules. After birth the baby can have breast engorgement due to withdrawal of oestrogens previously obtained in utero from its mother. Milk may form and sometimes can be expressed from the nipples, now slight prominences on the skin.

At puberty, the breasts enlarge under the influence of ovarian hormones, more ducts and glands being formed, but full development awaits a pregnancy and lactation.

In the adult, the mammary glands (breasts) lie between the 2nd and 6th rib, from the sternum to the axillary line. They consist largely of fat and connective tissue and are superficial to the pectoral muscles. The active tissue contains acinous glands from which ducts lead to the sinus lactiferous, from where 15–20 ducts pass to the nipple and exterior. At the base of the nipple is the areola, with muscle tissue and sebaceous Montgomery's tubercles which secrete a lubricant. The internal mammary blood vessels supply the mammary glands; lymph draining into the axillary glands.

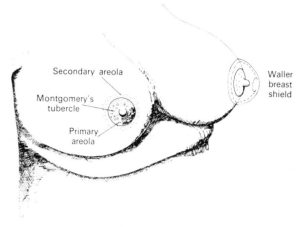

Secondary areola

Montgomery's
tubercle

Primary
areola

Waller
breast
shield

FIG. 3.12 Breasts

Secretion of milk is influenced by both pituitary and ovarian hormones but the main stimulation is by a baby's suction. Human breast milk differs in many ways from cow's milk. There is a relative difference in the quantity of calcium and phosphorus. Human milk contains important lysozymes which help to prevent infection. After delivery human milk takes a few weeks to becomes mature. The early secretion (colostrum) is yellow and contains easily digested protein; as the milk matures the colour changes. There is no doubt that human milk is the natural, ideal milk for the human baby during the first few months of life. In addition lactation is advantageous to the mother. Breast-feeding aids involution of the uterus, so that when menstruation recommences the blood loss should not be excessive.

There is some evidence that a breast-fed baby is less likely to develop coronary artery disease in adolescence. (Osborn, G. K. *in* Colloques Internationaux du Centre National de la Recherche Scientifique, No. 169, Paris, 1967.)

4   THE FETUS

Normally, in utero, the fetus is completely flexed and so occupies the minimum of space. The long fetal axis should correspond to the long axis of the uterus, giving a 'longitudinal' lie.

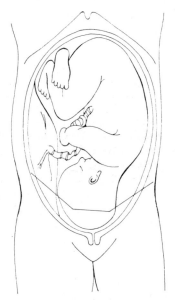

FIG. 4.1 Longitudinal lie of the fetus

The largest part of the fetus is the head and if this can traverse the pelvis the rest of the body normally follows easily. The fetal skull is therefore important in midwifery.

THE FETAL SKULL

The base does not really concern midwives, the vault is all important. This consists of two parietal bones, two frontal bones and the occiput.

The parietal bones are separated by the sagittal suture and join the occiput at the posterior fontanelle, but from there the lambdoid sutures pass laterally—this means that the posterior fontanelle is a small depressed membranous area with three sutures passing to it; it is triangular in shape.

Anteriorly, the parietal bones meet the two frontal bones at a much wider fontanelle—the anterior or Bregma—into this four sutures pass, i.e. the sagittal, the coronals separating the parietal from the frontal bones and the frontal suture.

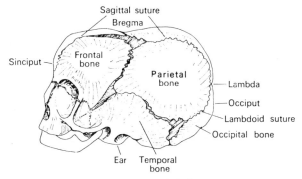

FIG. 4.2 Foetal skull

This fontanelle is reasonably large, covered by membrane making a distinct impression to the examining finger and is diamond-shaped.

In labour, the degree of flexion of the fetal skull determines which diameter of the fetal head encounters the pelvic diameters.

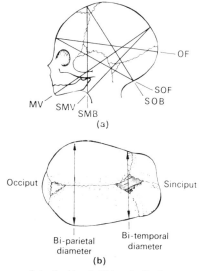

FIG. 4.3 Diameters of the fetal head: (a) longitudinal: MV = mento-vertical; SMV = submento-vertical; OF = occipito-frontal; SOF = suboccipito-frontal; SMB = submento-bregmatic; SOB = suboccipito-bregmatic. (b) transverse

A well-flexed head, as in occipito-anterior position, enables the suboccipito-bregmatic diameter (9·5 cm) to engage (i.e. enter the pelvis). A slightly less flexed head in a breech delivery means that the suboccipital-frontal diameter (10 cm) will engage. When the occiput is posterior the occipito-frontal diameter (11 cm) engages. If the fetal head is fully extended, the face presents (comes first) and the submento (under the chin)-bregmatic diameter (9·5 cm) engages.

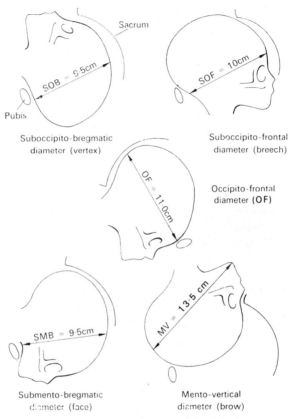

FIG. 4.4 Degrees of deflection of foetal head

A slightly less extended head means that the brow (sinciput) comes first and a large diameter, the mento-vertical (13·5 cm), presents.

Thus far, longitudinal measurements only of the fetal skull have been mentioned. Transversely, the widest part is between the parietal bone eminences, 9·5 cm. The next widest is lower than the vault between the temporal bones 8·5 cm.

The vertex is described as the area of skull between the anterior and posterior fontanelles. Considering the rest of the fetus—when the shoulders are born, the widest diameter is between the achromial processes, 10 cm, and (lower) at the buttocks, the bi-trochanteric, 10 cm.

When the bi-parietal diameter of the fetal skull has passed through the pelvic inlet, the fetal head is said to have engaged. The occiput will then be at the level of the ischial spines, and it may not be possible to feel the fetal head on abdominal palpation. This seldom occurs before labour is established. In the past there has been some confusion in the term 'engaged'—when the vertex enters the pelvic brim, the head is fixed but not usually truly engaged.

Inside the skull the cerebral hemispheres are separated by a vertical fibrous membrane, the falx cerebri (superior tentorium). This is attached to the frontal and

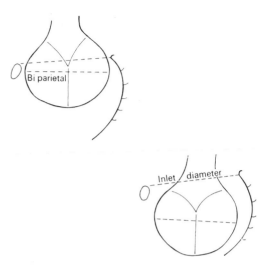

FIG. 4.5 Engagement of fetal head

sagittal sutures. Below a horizontal membrane, the tentorium cerebelli separates the cerebral hemispheres from the cerebellum and is attached to the occipital bone behind, but has a free edge in front. Excessive moulding of the fetal head during

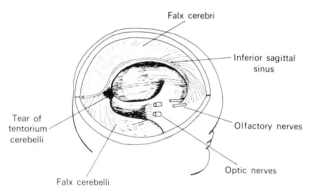

FIG. 4.6 Tentorial tears

labour can strain the junction between the two tentorii where the vein of Galen passes. If a tear should occur the fetus will suffer an intracranial haemorrhage and possible death. There is less strain on the tentorial junction when the fetal head is well flexed (occipito-anterior) than in an occipito-posterior presentation.

5 THE MENSTRUAL CYCLE

A female baby is born with typical female genitalia, but the labia are small. The labia develop before puberty and then hair appears at the mons pubis.

At birth the ovaries contain numerous primordial Graafian follicles which remain quiescent until the menarche (when menstruation begins). The menarche usually occurs about the age of 12–15 years. Growth of the labia and other secondary sexual characteristics is influenced by anterior pituitary hormones.

At the menarche, each month, one Graafian follicle matures. The follicle becomes cystic and the central nucleus (ovum) floats to the surface. The follicle rises to the

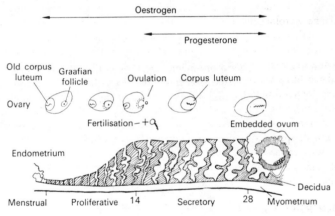

FIG. 5.1 Endometrial changes in the menstrual cycle

surface of the ovarian cortex and ruptures expelling the ovum (ovulation). The ovum is sucked into the fimbrial end of the neighbouring Fallopian tube. Unless the ovum meets a male spermatozoon, the ovum is wafted into the uterine cavity by the action of the ciliated epithelium lining the Fallopian tube. From the uterus the ovum is expelled through the cervix and vagina to the exterior. The ovum is one of the largest single cells of the body and is just visible to the naked eye. Usually, the ovum will have reached the vulva within 48 hours of leaving the ovary. With ovulation there is a slight rise of the body temperature.

Whilst the Graafian follicle matures, oestrogens are secreted from the covering granulosa cells. After ovulation the follicle changes into the corpus luteum. The covering granulosa cells become irregular in shape forming thecal cells. The follicle becomes haemorrhagic and acquires a yellow pigment. The thecal cells secrete progesterone. Unless the ovum has met a spermatozoon the corpus luteum degenerates into a corpus accreta, and ends as a slight scar on the ovarian cortex.

Menstruation

The cyclical ovarian changes affect the endometrium (lining mucous membrane of the uterus). Oestrogens stimulate growth of the endometrial cells; progesterone increases their blood supply and enables the endometrial cells to secrete glycogen. When the corpus luteum degenerates the entire endometrium is shed with some bleeding. This bleeding is termed *menstruation*. Bleeding usually occurs about every 28 days, lasting for 4–7 days. It is difficult to estimate the normal amount of bleeding. The loss should not lower the woman's haemoglobin or affect her general health. Usually 2 sanitary pads are required for the first 2 days and require to be changed about every 4 hours during the day. Nowadays an internal tampon is commonly used. This again requires to be replaced every 4 hours. After 48 hours the bleeding lessens. During menstruation slight abdominal discomfort is common but real pain (dysmenorrhoea) is abnormal. The passage of blood clots is abnormal. The first day of bleeding constitutes the beginning of the menstrual cycle. Ovulation usually occurs about the 10th–14th day. At this time there may be slight breast discomfort and some excess vaginal secretion. The temperature rises slightly. Some women have prolonged menstrual cycles, i.e. bleeding only occurring about every 35 days. In these cases the first follicular phase is lengthened and ovulation is late.

Menstruation ceases about the age of 45–55 years—the menopause. Thereafter the genital organs retrogress, no bleeding or ovulation occurring. This 'climacteric' period may be associated with hot flushes and headaches, but these symptoms should only last for a few months.

A woman can only conceive during her menstrual phase. During each cycle there is only a short fertile period after ovulation. For a pregnancy to occur the ovum must meet a male spermatozoon in a Fallopian tube. At intercourse the male inserts numerous spermatozoa from his seminal fluid into the vagina. Spermatozoa are mobile and can pass up through a healthy cervix into the uterine cavity and reach the Fallopian tubes, provided they are patent and healthy.

ENDOCRINE GLANDS

This is a complex subject as so many of these glands are inter-related. The key gland is probably the pituitary, lying in the skull at the base of the brain, close to the hypothalamus. The pituitary has an anterior and posterior lobe, each producing important hormones.

Posterior pituitary hormones

These include:

(1) *Pitressin* which is a factor in controlling blood pressure.

(2) *Pitocin* which causes a pregnant uterus to contract and during labour, retract.

Anterior pituitary hormones

These are numerous, including:

(1) *Growth hormone* which also causes the development of secondary sexual characteristics.

(2) *Diuretic hormone* affecting urinary output.

(3) *Insulin antagonising hormone* which influences blood sugar levels.

(4) *Prolactin* which stimulates milk secretion from the breasts in the puerperium.

(5) *Relaxin* which causes the ureters to dilate, and the pelvic joints to relax during pregnancy.

(6) *Gonadotrophic hormones* which stimulate the ovaries after the menarche. The gonadotrophic hormones include:

> (*a*) A follicular stimulating hormone (FSH) which causes a Graafian follicle to ripen and expel an ovum.
>
> (b) A luteal hormone (LH) which controls the development of the corpus luteum.

During pregnancy gonadotrophic hormones are excreted in the urine.

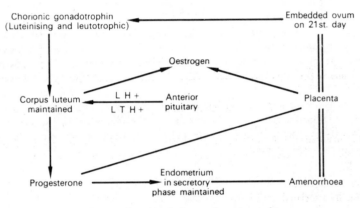

FIG. 5.2 Anterior pituitary and ovarian cycle

Other Endocrine Glands

(1) *Suprarenals* situated above each kidney. The suprarenal gland consists of a cortex and medulla. The cortex produces hormones which control the salt and water balance in the body cells, and melanin which affects pigmentation. From the medulla, adrenaline is produced which stimulates voluntary muscles.

(2) *Thyroid gland.* This is bilobular, lying anterior to the trachea, but a portion can be behind the sternum. This gland requires iodine to function and enlarges during pregnancy. Thyroid hormones control general metabolism.

(3) *Thymus gland.* This is relatively large in a newborn baby and is now thought to be important in immunology. The thymus gland lies behind the sternum.

(4) *The Pancreas* produces insulin which controls the absorption of glucose, also trypsin which is essential for protein digestion.

(5) *Ovarian hormones*

> (a) *Oestrogens* are produced during the follicular ovarian phase. The effect of oestrogens on the uterine endometrium is described under menstruation.
>
> Oestrogens are essential for the maintenance of pregnancy but may be produced by the placenta and fetus. Like other hormones, oestrogens circulate in the bloodstream and undergo chemical changes in the liver before excretion

by the kidneys as oestriol. The quantity excreted during pregnancy can indicate placental function, a fall suggesting that the fetus is at risk.

(b) *Progesterone* is produced during the luteal ovarian phase and is essential for

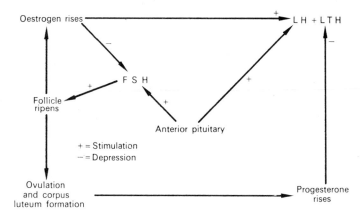

FIG. 5.3 Hormonal changes in pregnancy

the maintenance of pregnancy. The relative quantities of oestrogen and progesterone can be determined by microscopic examination of vaginal epithelial cells.

(c) *Androgen* (male hormone) is also secreted by the ovaries. Excess androgen is usually associated with hirsutism (male characteristics).

6 FERTILISATION AND FETAL DEVELOPMENT

FERTILISATION

Fertilisation occurs when a male spermatozoon meets an ovum. This usually occurs in the outer third of a Fallopian tube. The sperm and ovum both shed half their chromosomes, so that the fertilised ovum contains 46 chromosomes. These are responsible for genetic characteristics, determining sex, blood group etc. Regarding sex, a female carries XX chromosomes, the male XY. Therefore the sex of the fetus really depends on which chromosome X or Y the sperm sheds. Unless the chromosome number remains at 46 after fertilisation, the fetus may be abnormal.

Development of the Fertilised Ovum

After fertilisation the two cells multiply rapidly into a morula. This passes along the Fallopian tube to the uterine cavity because of the action of the ciliated epithelium lining the tube. In the uterus glycogen produced by the decidua (exaggerated

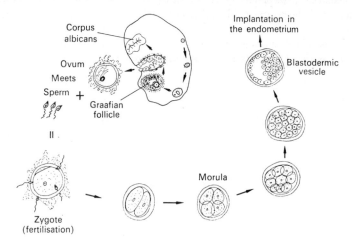

FIG. 6.1 Ovulation and fertilisation with early embryonic development

progesterone type of endometrium) nourishes the morula for a short period. Soon the solid morula becomes cystic, the cells being pushed together as the inner cell mass and fluid collects. Now the structure is called a blastodermic vesicle. The outer covering branches from a smooth membrane into the trophoblast. This is capable of digesting its way into the decidua, usually near the upper part of the uterus. After embedding, the uterine opening is sealed off. The trophoblast branches into chorionic villi. Some villi anchor the blastocyst to the base of the decidua but should not

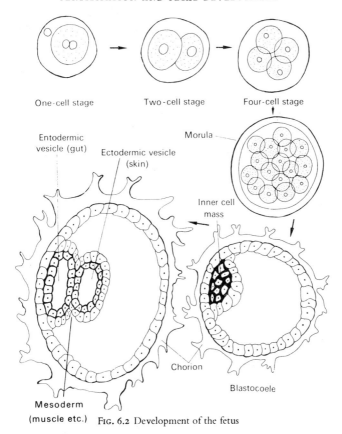

One-cell stage   Two-cell stage   Four-cell stage

Entodermic
vesicle (gut)   Ectodermic vesicle
                       (skin)

Morula

Inner cell
mass

Chorion

Blastocoele

Mesoderm
(muscle etc.)   FIG. 6.2 Development of the fetus

penetrate into muscle; others penetrate into maternal blood vessels forming sinuses. The trophoblast consists of a double cellular membrane, the syncytium and the layer of Langhans. The basal villi continue to develop forming part of the placenta;

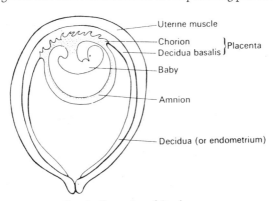

Uterine muscle

Chorion
Decidua basalis }Placenta

Baby

Amnion

Decidua (or endometrium)

FIG. 6.3 Formation of the placenta

surrounding villi become superfluous and degenerate into a smooth membrane, the chorion.

Development of the Fetus

The inner cell mass develops into the fetus. Nourishment passes out of the blood in the maternal uterine blood sinuses, and is absorbed through the chorionic villi double cellular layer into the fetal blood. This flows along a circular sinus in the chorion passing to the fetus via a broad primitive body stalk. Uterine contractions aid this primitive circulation.

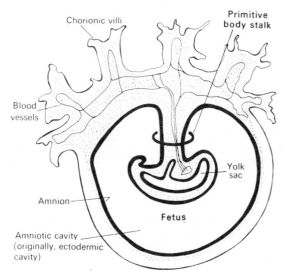

FIG. 6.4 Circulation in the embryo

After it is embedded, the fetus grows rapidly, and soon the surfaces of the uterus are pushed together and the potential uterine cavity is closed. Embryonic development of the inner cell mass is spectacularly rapid and complex. Ectoderm, mesoderm and endoderm tissues produce skin tissues, muscle and internal organs respectively.

Four weeks from ovulation the fetal shape resembles a mammal and is 1 cm long. A tail is obvious—the ventral stalk is inserted into the umbilicus but intestines may be present in the cord. By 8 weeks limbs have developed. At 12 weeks the fetus is obviously human and the external genitalia reveal the sex. The length now is 9 cm. All essential organs form before the 12th week. After this the fetus continues to grow. Its length is described in cm (lunar months squared) until the 28th week. At this time the fetus is said to be viable, i.e. if born the fetus attempts to breathe. After 28 weeks the length is usually recorded in inches (the weeks divided by half) i.e. at 28 weeks the fetus is 36 cm long, at 40 weeks, 20 inches (50 cm). After 28 weeks the fetal muscles develop and fat is laid down. The fetus is covered by fine lanugo hair and coated with a greasy substance, vernix. The fetus

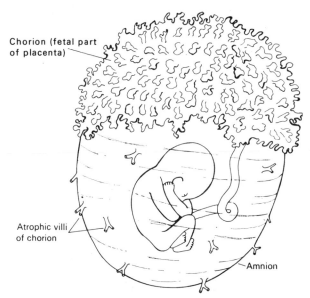

Chorion (fetal part of placenta)

Atrophic villi of chorion

Amnion

FIG. 6.5 Fetus at the fourth month

in developing requires freedom of movement; therefore from the inner cell mass the amniotic cells develop and form the amniotic cavity. The amnion is firmly adherent to the fetal ventral stalk and closely applied to the chorion.

Amniotic fluid is produced partly by absorption from the maternal circulation through the amniotic cells and partly by fetal urine. The amniotic cells produce vernix and probably oestrogens. Amniotic fluid is swallowed by the fetus and some passes into the fetal lungs.

THE PLACENTA

The placenta is formed by the time the fetus is 12 weeks old. The maternal surface consists of decidua, with chorionic villi attached to the decidua and other villi, which have penetrated into the maternal blood vessels, producing sinuses.

At term the placenta is a haemorrhagic structure with two surfaces, the maternal and fetal. The placenta resembles a flat pancake approximately 30·5 cm in diameter and about 2·5 cm in depth at the centre. The weight averages 1½ lbs (680 g) but in process of development the placental weight should bear a close relation to the fetal weight, usually about one-sixth. The maternal surface is covered by a greyish membrane, the decidua. Beneath this the chorionic villi produce cotyledons divided by fissures or sulci. At the edge the chorionic membrane is firmly adherent, but round the edge there may be remnants of the early fetal circulatory sinus. The fetal surface is lined by the amnion with the smooth chorion beneath. Blood vessels from the umbilical cord usually enter the placenta near the centre, thereafter dividing and penetrating into the placental cotyledons.

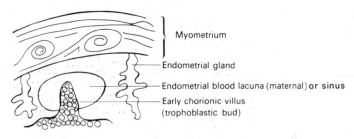

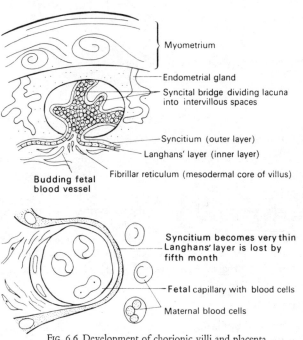

Fig. 6.6 Development of chorionic villi and placenta

Several varieties of placenta are recognised:

(1) *Battledore.* The cord is inserted into the placenta near its circumference.

(2) *Velamentous.* The cord ends in membrane and divided blood vessels then proceed to the placenta.

(3) *Subchorionic.* The circular sinus remains as a thickened structure preventing the normal expansion of the placental diameter. The villi have to grow beneath this ridge. This type of placenta used to be called circumvallate.

(4) *Succenturiate.* An additional placental lobe can develop in the chorionic membrane away from the main placental mass. This type is usual in certain animals, e.g. the cow. Blood vessels from the placenta pass in the membrane to the additional lobe. A succenturiate lobe is often abnormally adherent to the uterine wall.

(5) *Bi- or tri-lobular.* Occasionally the placenta instead of being a roughly circular shape is lobulated—this does not appear to be of any significance.

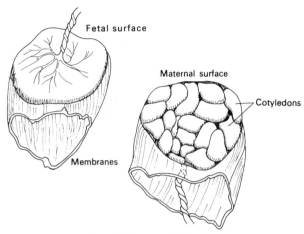

FIG. 6.7 The normal placenta

Functions of the Placenta

(1) *Nutritive.* The fetus acquires all nutrition from uterine blood vessels through the placenta. Maternal and fetal blood does not mix directly because of the membranes covering the chorionic villi.

(2) *Respiratory.* Oxygen is obtained from the uterine arteries and carbon dioxide is expelled through the placenta into the uterine veins.

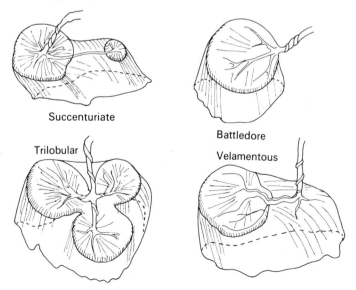

FIG. 6.8 Varieties of placenta

(3) *Barrier Action*. Bacilli usually fail to pass through the chorionic membrane, but viruses can pass through. Drugs also pass. Some organisms, e.g. syphilitic spirochaetes, attack the placental tissue and break down the barrier between fetal and maternal blood supplies.

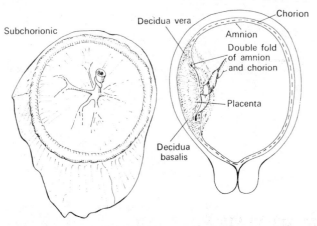

FIG. 6.9 Subchorionic (circumvallate) placenta

(4) *Endocrine*. The placenta secretes ovarian hormones and stores them.
(5) *Storage*. Glycogen, and possibly other nutritive substances are stored in the placenta.

The Umbilical Cord

This develops from the primitive ventral stalk and is attached to the fetal umbilicus and passes to the placenta.

At term the average length of the umbilical cord is 50·5 cm; a shorter cord may give rise to early placental separation and an excessively long cord may twist around the fetus or prolapse when the membranes rupture during labour.

The umbilical cord consists of a primitive connective tissue, Wharton's jelly. Sometimes this produces thickened lumps commonly known as 'fasle knots'. Within the cord are vital blood vessels and the Wharton's jelly prevents compression of these vessels. At term the cord contains two arteries and one vein (although early in fetal life two veins are present). Occasionally, one artery is absent and this may occur when the fetus is abnormal, e.g. renal agenesis. The vessels are spiral, i.e. twisted around one another. The thickness of the umbilical cord varies with the quantity of Wharton's jelly.

If the cord is abnormally thin, compression of the cord vessels tends to occur. Occasionally, especially when the cord is unduly long, a true knot is found, presumably because the fetus has twisted the cord during excessive activity. The amniotic membrane is closely attached to the umbilical cord. Early in fetal life some loops of intestine are contained in the primitive umbilical cord, but these are rarely still there at birth.

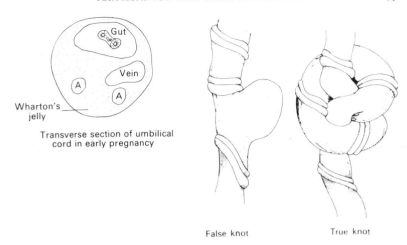

Wharton's jelly

Transverse section of umbilical
cord in early pregnancy

False knot

True knot

FIG. 6.10 Abnormalities of the umbilical cord

FETAL CIRCULATION

The fetus at term has the normal four heart cavities—two ventricles and two atria. There is a communication between the atria, the foramen ovale, which should close shortly after birth. From the right ventricle the pulmonary artery communicates directly with the aorta via the ductus arteriosus, and this also closes shortly after birth.

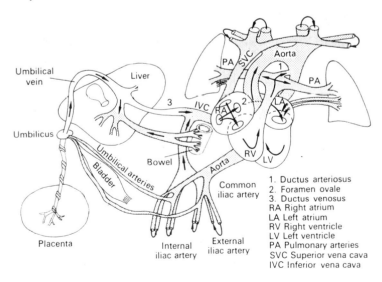

1. Ductus arteriosus
2. Foramen ovale
3. Ductus venosus
RA Right atrium
LA Left atrium
RV Right ventricle
LV Left ventricle
PA Pulmonary arteries
SVC Superior vena cava
IVC Inferior vena cava

FIG. 6.11 Diagram of the fetal circulation. Arrows show direction of flow,
shading denotes degree of oxygenation

Deoxygenated blood passes from the hypogastric arteries (branches of the internal iliac arteries) into the umbilical cord and, after oxygenisation in the placenta, pure blood passes via the umbilical vein through the inferior vena cava (communicating with the liver) to the right auricle. Most of the blood will pass through the foramen ovale to the left atrium, thence to the left ventricle and aorta to be distributed to the abdomen and lower limbs. Some will pass from the right atrium to the right ventricle and via the pulmonary artery to the lungs, but as these barely function in utero, the majority is diverted via the ductus arteriosus to the aorta.

At birth, when the lungs expand, there are pressure changes in the heart chambers which induce closure of the foramen ovale and ductus arteriosus.

7 BLOOD GROUPS

The blood group of an individual is determined early in fetal life and depends on blood factors inherited from both the sperm and ovum, i.e. father and mother. The ABO group factors are important, an individual having only A (group A), only B (group B), both A and B (group AB) or neither A nor B (group O).

The CDE/cde factors form another important group and many combinations are obviously possible. Any individual having one 'D' is known as heterozygous Rhesus (Rh) positive, with two 'D's' homozygous Rhesus (Rh) positive. The individual with two 'd's' is Rhesus negative.

Patients with, for example, group O (lacking A and B factors) may react if they receive blood of a group other than their own. The same is true when the patient is Rhesus negative and receives Rh positive, especially D, blood.

Heredity of the Rhesus Factor

'D' is dominant; 'd' is recessive.

A Rhesus negative woman (♀) is 'dd'—i.e. homozygous.
A Rhesus positive man (♂) is either 'DD' (= homozygous) or 'Dd' (= heterozygous).

Possibilities of Offspring

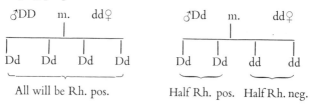

During pregnancy, women who may be carrying a fetus with a blood group differing from their own are vulnerable. In a normal pregnancy, fetal and maternal blood seldom mix but during delivery, mixture will occur. The blood group which is unnatural to the mother causes sensitisation and later antibodies can develop. Mixing of fetal and maternal blood is especially liable to occur during abnormal labours, e.g. at the time of a Caesarean Section or where the placenta has to be separated manually.

Haemolytic Disease

When sensitisation has occurred, antibodies can develop and affect the fetus during a subsequent pregnancy, causing *haemolytic disease*. Fetal blood cells are broken down, causing fetal anaemia. In severe cases, the fetus will die in utero, or the fetus will be born with hydrops due to cardiac failure. In less severe cases, the baby will become jaundiced and anaemic within 48 hours of birth. A severe jaundice affects the basal ganglia and can cause kernicterus, resulting in a spastic or sub-mentally developed child.

Obstetricians and midwives must strive to prevent haemolytic disease of the newborn.

Prevention of Haemolytic Disease

(1) No unnecessary blood transfusions should be given. Their need will be reduced if anaemia is diagnosed and treated prior to labour. If transfusion becomes necessary, only blood similar in grouping should be given, careful cross-matching being necessary; to be efficient this may require 3 hours.

(2) The blood group of every pregnant woman must be determined. Provided she is Rhesus positive and not group O, there is no need to repeat tests during subsequent pregnancies. The patient will have a card issued from the blood transfusion centre. Each group has a separate colour.

If the mother is group O Rhesus positive, it is advisable to test her blood during each pregnancy in case the fetal blood contains A or B factors.

If the mother is Rhesus D negative, it is essential for her to have repeated blood tests during pregnancy. These tests are usually performed early in pregnancy, again about the 29th week and between the 34th–36th week. Only a small per-centage of women will produce antibodies.

(3) If antibodies are detected during pregnancy, the woman must be delivered in hospital under consultant care.

The husband's blood should be grouped. In cases of Rh D immunisation, the husband may be either homozygous Rh positive (when the baby will of necessity be Rh D positive), or heterozygous. If the latter, 50 per cent of the fetuses will be Rh negative and unaffected.

(4) First babies are seldom affected, unless the mother has received incompatible blood. The number of fetal cells in the maternal circulation after delivery can be assessed. This should be done in primipara who are Rhesus D negative. Sensitisation to the Rhesus factor is more likely when the baby's ABO group is identical to the mother's.

A sample of cord blood will be necessary to determine the baby's ABO group and also the Rhesus factor.

Antibody formation to the Rh D factor can be prevented by giving immune anti D globulin to the mother within 60 hours of delivery. Because of limited supplies, anti D globulin was only given when the first child was of the same ABO group as the mother and Rh positive. With a second child anti D globulin was only given when the presence of fetal blood cells had been found in the maternal blood after delivery.

Supplies of anti D globulin have increased. Since July 1971 all Rhesus negative women who give birth to a Rhesus positive baby, regardless of parity or ABO group should be given 100 μg Anti D globulin. If there are a considerable number of fetal cells in the maternal blood the dose of anti D globulin should be doubled.

Rhesus negative women having a therapeutic abortion should receive 50 μg Anti D globulin unless sterilisation is also done.

(5) When antibodies, especially anti-D, are detected in a pregnant woman's blood, fetal prognosis can be determined by the past history of her babies, by the antibody

titre and also by examining the liquor amnii spectroscopically. This is obtained by abdominal paracentesis.

Optimum results require expert obstetrical and paediatric decisions. In severe cases, where there is a grave risk of fetal death prior to the 33rd week, intra-uterine peritoneal blood infusions can be given. This involves elaborate technique and good results will only be possible in specialised units.

Between the 34th–36th weeks, delivery by Caesarean Section may be advisable. After the 36th week, vaginal delivery following surgical induction of labour gives the best result.

Jaundice will be more severe if the baby has to be born prematurely because a premature baby's liver is immature.

(6) When antibodies have been detected, a sample of cord blood must be taken to determine the baby's blood group, haemoglobin level and bilirubin. This sample should be collected before placental separation, otherwise haemolysis is likely.

The baby may require an exchange blood transfusion in order to prevent severe jaundice and the transfusion may have to be repeated if the baby's bilirubin rises to a high level (20–25 mg). The paediatrician gives the transfusion through the umbilical vein; therefore at birth the umbilical cord should be divided not less than 5 cm from the umbilicus. Later the baby may require a blood transfusion for anaemia.

With the use of phototherapy and phenobarbitone, the level of bilirubin falls and fewer exchange blood transfusions are required.

8 PHYSIOLOGY AND DIAGNOSIS OF PREGNANCY

PHYSIOLOGY OF PREGNANCY

The Uterus

The uterus is the chief organ to be altered during pregnancy. As soon as the fertilised ovum embeds in the uterine decidua, the uterus has to expand. The uterus softens and becomes globular in shape, and three distinct muscle layers develop. The involuntary muscles contract and relax (Braxton Hick's contractions). This squeezes blood from the maternal uterine blood sinuses, through the primitive chorionic vessels, to supply the developing fetus and return fetal waste products. At first the contractions are infrequent, every 20–30 minutes. Therefore if a doctor makes a vaginal examination early in pregnancy, the contractions may or may not be felt. Pulsating vessels in the vaginal fornices are a more constant finding. The cervix and uterus feel soft.

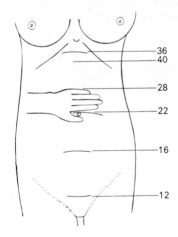

FIG. 8.1 Gestational height of the fundus calculated in weeks

With growth the uterus rises into the abdomen and by the 12th week the uterine fundus can be felt above the symphysis pubis, often earlier in a multipara. Growth in a normal single pregnancy is remarkably constant. By the 22nd week the fundus reaches the umbilicus, provided this is in the normal position (halfway between the symphysis pubis and xiphisternum). By the 36th week the fundus reaches the upper limits of the abdomen. If the fetal head engages at this stage, as is usual in a primigravida, little further uterine expansion is necessary. However, if the fetal head remains free, further uterine expansion is forwards, overstretching the anterior abdominal wall causing the abdomen to appear pendulous. When the uterus rises out of the pelvis the uterine appendages (Fallopian tubes and ovaries) rise also and become abdominal organs. This entails growth of the broad and round ligaments. Uterine blood vessels multiply to nourish the expanding uterus and contents. At term the uterus weighs approximately 964 g, its length averages 30·5 cm, width 23 cm and depth 20 cm; its wall is slightly thinner than in a non-pregnant uterus.

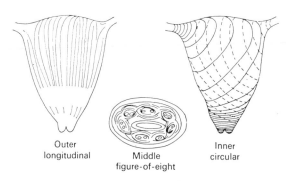

Outer longitudinal Middle figure-of-eight Inner circular

FIG. 8.2 Musculature of the uterus

With growth of the uterus the active longitudinal muscles form a distinct upper uterine segment differentiated from the lower passive segment, including the cervix. This latter passive portion is under sympathetic voluntary muscle control. The junction between the two segments is shown by the peritoneum which is firmly adherent to the upper active segment but loosely applied to the lower segment, because the peritoneum passes forwards to the bladder.

The Cervix

During pregnancy the cervical glands and their nuclei are very active. Extra secretion of mucus softens the cervix so that it is ready to stretch during labour. An extra blood supply makes the vaginal portion of the cervix take on a violet colour.

The Vagina

Vaginal epithelial cells alter with ovarian hormones (oestrogen and progesterone). During pregnancy particularly, a vaginal smear may determine the relative activity of these hormones (cornification index). The acidity of the vaginal mucosa falls in pregnancy and this makes the vagina vulnerable to infection. Increased vascularity gives the vulva a violet tinge, noticeable only after a few months.

The Ovaries

When an ovary has expelled an ovum which becomes fertilised, the corpus luteum, instead of degenerating, remains active for at least 12 weeks, producing progesterone. After this time the placenta seems to 'take over' this hormone production. With the prolonged action of progesterone menstrual bleeding ceases throughout pregnancy.

The Breasts

During pregnancy additional glands and ducts are formed. Quite early, extra blood circulates and the pregnant woman may complain of 'tingling' in the breasts. The nipples develop, becoming more erect; they are lubricated by the increased activity of Montgomery's tubercles (sebaceous glands). A brown pigmentation of the areoli occurs early (primary areoli). Later a patchy pigmentation may surround the skin outside the areolar area (secondary areola). These pigmentary changes are more pronounced in brunettes. In the later weeks of pregnancy colostrum can often be expressed from the nipples and sometimes leaks spontaneously.

Maternal Systems in Pregnancy

All maternal organs work harder than usual during pregnancy and the various systems will be described.

Circulatory

During pregnancy the blood volume increases, reaching a maximum between the 28th and 36th week. This increase requires the formation of extra blood cells and haemoglobin, which means that additional iron is needed to prevent anaemia. Some iron, however, is conserved owing to the absence of menstrual bleeding. The heart works harder than usual. Its apex is pushed to the left and there are some pressure changes in the heart chambers. Praecordial murmurs are common. A normal heart has adequate reserve power for pregnancy, but if a woman has a cardiac lesion pregnancy can precipitate failure.

The blood pressure tends to fall when the blood volume increases. Maximum normal levels, during pregnancy, should not exceed 130 systolic and 80 diastolic. Owing to increased abdominal pressure pregnancy may cause or aggravate varicose veins in the lower limbs and at the vulva and anus (haemorrhoids). The veins, however, seldom thrombose, which suggests that blood clots less readily during pregnancy. The exact reason for this is not known, but it may protect the placental circulation.

Respiratory

In pregnancy additional oxygen is required for the fetus, and the fetal carbon dioxide has also to be removed by the maternal lungs. When the diaphragm rises, as it does in late pregnancy, the circumference of the chest expands so that the volume of the pleural cavities remain normal.

Urinary

In order to deal with fetal waste products and extra maternal metabolites, the maternal kidneys perform about 30 per cent additional work. Normal kidneys have reserve power but diseased kidneys may fail. The ureters dilate under the action of relaxin. The ureters may be compressed at the pelvic brim, especially on the right side, and compression leads to stasis of urine and liability to infection. Thus pyelitis or pyelonephritis are common complications of pregnancy.

In the early weeks of pregnancy, when the pelvic uterus is growing, the bladder may be compressed causing frequency of micturition. The same may occur towards the end of pregnancy when the fetal head engages.

Alimentary

Nausea or actual vomiting in the morning is common in early pregnancy, but usually ceases by the 12th week. Alteration in hormone balance may be the cause by lowering the blood sugar. Occasionally excessive salivation occurs without known cause, again early in pregnancy. Later in pregnancy the stomach may be compressed and produce less than its normal amount of pepsin and hydrochloric acid and the cardiac sphincter may relax. This can cause indigestion. If a pregnant woman has a hiatus hernia, her symptoms are aggravated during late pregnancy.

The liver (a vital organ) works extra hard and is very susceptible to damage through drugs and infection. Constipation should not occur if the diet contains adequate roughage. Haemorrhoids can be a nuisance.

Skeletal

In the upright position the pregnant abdomen puts a strain on the lumbar vertebrae. In compensation the pregnant woman tends to hold her head upright (the 'pride of pregnancy') and braces her shoulders back. The pelvic joints, especially late in pregnancy, soften and widen. Occasionally this is excessive causing pain on walking (pelvic arthropathy).

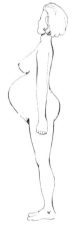

FIG. 8.3 'Pride of pregnancy'

The Skin

Striae (stretch marks) are common on the abdominal skin, sometimes on the buttocks, outer thighs and over the mammary glands. Striae are pink lines varying in length from 1·25 cm–5 cm, which afterwards fade to white but do not disappear. According to a modern theory the cause is more hormonal (progesterone) than sheer tension. Pregnancy stimulates the formation of extra melanin. This causes the linea nigra (brown line from the umbilicus to the symphysis pubis). Recent abdominal operation scars are darkened. Melanin also accounts for breast pigmentation. Sometimes excessive freckling of the face occurs (cloasma). During pregnancy skin rashes are common, probably due to altered blood chemistry. These rashes can be difficult to cure.

Nervous

Pregnancy is an exciting experience. Fear of the unknown and particularly 'old wives' tales' may create fright. Mental instability may become manifest, although true psychosis occurs more commonly after the child has been born. Neurosis may cause abnormal food dislikes and prevent an optimal diet. Pregnant women require sympathy and understanding.

Recently psychiatrists have suggested that potential fathers are also under mental tension.

Endocrine

All endocrine glands produce extra hormones during pregnancy. This can cause a noticeable enlargement of the thyroid gland; an abnormal blood sugar curve can arise and potential diabetes become manifest. Ovarian hormones (oestrogens and progesterone) are essential for the maintenance of pregnancy. An excessive amount of pituitary (gonadotrophin) hormone is excreted in the urine.

Weight

The average weight gain in pregnancy is $1\frac{1}{2}$ stone (9·5 kg), more than can be accounted for by the fetal weight, placenta and liquor amnii. Some of this gain is due to fluid retention and some to fat deposition. The main weight gain occurs between the 12th and 36th week, but should never exceed 1 lb (879 g) in any one week.

Quickening

This term describes the first time that a pregnant woman becomes aware of fetal life (or fluttering). This usually occurs around the 18th week.

Length of Pregnancy

The expected date of confinement (EDC) is usually calculated as 40 weeks from the 1st day of the last menstrual period. A quick reckoning is to add one year, subtract three months and then add one week. If the pregnant woman can tell the exact date of conception from intercourse, 38 weeks is the average length of pregnancy assuming that she normally has a 28-day menstrual cycle. Only 3 per cent of women will be delivered on the exact date calculated for confinement. Seventy five per cent will be delivered in the preceding or succeeding week.

Diagnosis of Pregnancy

Positive signs of pregnancy do not occur until its latter half.
These are:

(1) Feeling fetal parts
(2) Hearing a fetal heart
(3) Seeing the fetus by X-ray
(4) Feeling the fetus move.

Earlier one is dependent on the patient's history (symptoms) and these symptoms only mean that pregnancy is a possibility and there are other possibilities. The symptoms are:

(1) Amenorrhoea (cessation of menstrual periods)
(2) Nausea or vomiting in the morning
(3) Tingling in the breasts
(4) Frequency of micturition without pain.

Early presumptive signs of pregnancy may be apparent on a vaginal examination by a doctor. A soft, large uterus may be felt and a soft cervix with pulsation in the fornices and possibly uterine contractions. After 12 weeks amenorrhoea, a central lower abdominal swelling suggests a pregnancy. Some laboratory tests are helpful but not fool-proof. The urine in pregnancy contains excessive gonadotrophin hormones and these are most pronounced in the first urine passed in the morning. Originally such a specimen was injected into a suitable non-pregnant female animal—at first a mouse (Zondek–Aschheim test), later a rabbit (Friedman test). This entailed examinations of the animal's ovaries to look for a corpus luteum, so the animal had to be killed. To prevent this, Hogben used a South African toad in which the urinary hormone stimulated ovulation with extrusion of egg cells. Nowadays animals are unnecessary since immunological laboratory tests have been devised.

9 ANTENATAL CARE

Aristotle (about 350 B.C.) spoke about the importance of diet and exercise in pregnancy. The first published work was by Thomas Bull in 1837. This was titled 'Hints to mothers for the management of health during the period of pregnancy and the lying-in room, with an exposure of the common errors in connection with these subjects.' In 1901 Ballantyne in Edinburgh suggested that there was a need for 'pre-maternity' beds in order to study antenatal pathology and reduce the number of still-births. During the same year in Boston, U.S.A. nurses were sent out from the Boston 'Lying-in' Hospital to visit pregnant women at home. Similar visiting was introduced in Edinburgh in 1913; the visit included recording the woman's blood pressure and obtaining a sample of urine which was tested for albumin. In 1915 the Simpson Maternity Hospital, Edinburgh, held antenatal clinics.

Antenatal care, in the true sense, was not established until the Public Health Act was passed in 1936. This Act put the onus onto Local Authorities to ensure adequate antenatal care, and Welfare Centres were set up. Since the introduction of the National Health Service in 1948, pregnant women have been able to receive antenatal care from three sources:

(1) Hospital, if booked for a hospital delivery
(2) Their own general practitioner
(3) Local Area Health Authority Clinics and/or domiciliary midwives.

A mother can attend all three, but this need not matter, provided each examination is recorded on a co-operation form, stating all advice and treatment given.

Nowadays regular antenatal examination is generally accepted by pregnant women. The reasons for this care are:

(1) Pregnancy strains all maternal organs. If previous existing disease, e.g. heart disease, can be recognised and treated, it may be possible to prevent serious consequences to both mother and baby.

(2) A healthy fetus requires nourishment and all essentials are obtained from the mother's diet.

(3) Pregnancy can give rise to various complications, e.g. toxaemia and various types of anaemia. Early recognition of these complications can usually preserve the health of the mother and baby.

(4) If a difficult labour can be anticipated (by recognising a malpresentation or diagnosing an abnormal pelvis), suitable preparations for labour can be made in good time.

(5) A simple explanation of labour, combined with relaxation exercises, reduces fear and renders labour less painful. This means that fewer pain-relieving drugs (analgesics) are required which is of advantage, since all such drugs are potentially dangerous to the fetus.

(6) Minor complications can worry a pregnant woman and simple advice can often help.

FIRST MEDICAL EXAMINATION

Antenatal care begins with a thorough medical examination, preferably early in pregnancy. This entails recording the patient's name, address, age, date of marriage (for fertility), race of herself and husband. If unmarried, the name and address of her nearest relative is noted. The husband's health and occupation are important to determine the social class. If the pregnant woman is working, this and the type of work should be noted. A full history is recorded of any previous medical or surgical illnesses. Any family history of twins, diabetes, hypertension, deafness or tuberculosis is noted. If the patient has already had children (a multipara) any abnormality during pregnancy, labour or after, must be recorded. The birth weight and maturity of each baby, with the birth date, is important. This obstetrical history must include miscarriages, still-births and babies who have died. It is important to ask the mother if she breast fed her babies.

It must be stressed that at this first interview the patient is often excited and nervous; the manner in which she is received and the way questions are asked are most important. The pregnant woman's confidence must be gained and kindness and sympathy expressed. It is necessary to stress that pregnancy is a natural phenomenon.

The menstrual history should be recorded, enquiring about the length and regularity of the periods. The first day of the last menstrual period is noted so that the approximate date for delivery can be calculated. In regard to the present pregnancy, suitable questions must be asked in order to confirm the probability of pregnancy and discover any complications. It is important to know if the patient is taking drugs, or has had, or been in contact with, virus infections, particularly rubella.

After questioning, the patient is asked to empty her bladder, the urine being collected into a suitable receiver. Various contraptions can be attached to a lavatory seat. The urine is tested for protein, glucose, pus and acetone (if the patient gives a history of vomiting).

The patient should next undress completely and don a lightweight dressing gown. Then her weight is recorded, also her height. Her gait is watched for any limp or evidence of rickets. She is asked to lie on an examination couch when the doctor endeavours to confirm pregnancy, if need be by a vaginal examination. Her breasts are palpated for any abnormality and the type of nipple noted. Evidence of hirsutism is looked for. The vulva is inspected for any abnormal vaginal discharge or previous perineal laceration. Her heart and lungs are auscultated. The blood pressure is recorded. Varicose veins are looked for.

A sample of blood is taken to determine the patient's haemoglobin. A sample is sent to an appropriate laboratory for testing to exclude syphilis. Unless the patient's blood group is known and she can produce her blood group card, a sample is sent to the blood transfusion centre. If she is rhesus negative or group O rhesus positive, a sample is sent to exclude antibodies.

All examinations should be explained to the patient and throughout she should be reassured.

Delivery and Discharge

After pregnancy has been established, the next decision to be made is where the patient should have her baby. Delivery in hospital is advisable in all the following cases:

(1) Young primigravidae (patients less than 20 years-old).
(2) Primigravidae over 28 years.
(3) Infertile women (i.e. a patient who has tried to conceive for 2½ years or more).
(4) Primigravidae less than 5 feet in height or showing evidence of hirsutism. (Ideally all primigravidae should be delivered in hospital.)
(5) Patients with any abnormal organ.
(6) Patients with previous obstetrical complications, e.g. toxaemia, previous complications during labour, especially haemorrhage, or any early puerperal abnormality.
(7) Any patient, whatever her parity, over the age of 35 years.
(8) Grand multiparae (4 or more previous deliveries).
(9) Rhesus negative women, pregnant for the first time or without a living child or with only one child.

Even when a normal confinement is anticipated complications can and do arise. Because of this risk, countries such as America and the Antipodean countries have encouraged all women to be delivered in hospital, either in a specialist unit or a fully equipped general practitioner maternity department. Britain is now following this pattern.

Multiparous patients may be anxious to return home early. After a normal labour, provided the baby's birth weight is at least 6 lb (2·7 kg) the patient need not remain in hospital for more than 48 hours. Such early discharge should be arranged with the area health authority during the pregnancy in order that a district midwife may visit the home, ensuring that adequate facilities are available for the care of a young baby and mother. After mother and baby have left hospital the domiciliary midwife will take over the puerperal treatment.

With a reduction in home deliveries domiciliary midwives are being encouraged to accompany 'early discharge' patients into hospital either into GP units or sometimes Specialist units, supervising a normal delivery and caring for the patient and baby prior to and after going home.

FURTHER MEDICAL EXAMINATIONS

All pregnant women should be advised to see a dentist (dental care is free in pregnancy).

All pregnant women until recently were encouraged to have a chest X-ray to exclude pulmonary tuberculosis; the optimum time is between the 14th and 26th week and the optimum place a mass radiography centre. There a large film is taken, screening off the abdomen and using a minimal X-ray dosage. Because, fortunately, the incidence of pulmonary tuberculosis in Britain has been reduced, the present recommendation by the Ministry of Health is to limit a chest X-ray during pregnancy to all women who have not had one done within 3 years, or within one year, if the patient lives in poor social conditions or is BCG negative or an immigrant.

In a normal pregnancy further examinations should be made as follows:
Every 4th week until the 28th week.
Every 2nd week until the 36th week.
Every week until delivered.

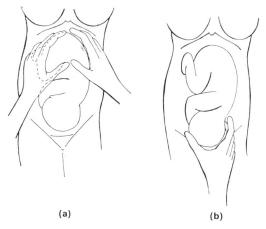

(a)   (b)

FIG. 9.1 Abdominal palpitation for (a) the fundus, (b) the head

Many of these examinations can be made by a midwife but she must seek medical
aid if any abnormality is suspected.

At each visit any complaint or anxieties of the patient must be noted. Her weight
and blood pressure are taken and the urine tested for protein and glucose. After the

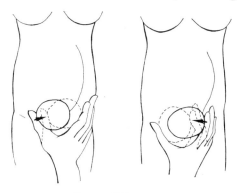

FIG. 9.2 Ballottement

12th week an abdominal examination is important. This examination begins with
inspection for any peculiar shape and is followed by palpation of the fundal height
to ascertain that this corresponds to the period of gestation. The lie and presentation
of the fetus should be determined after the 28th week and the fetal heart rate
noted. Warm hands and gentleness are necessary.

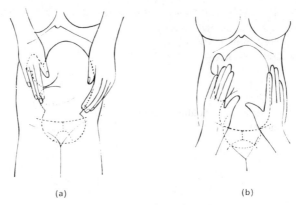

(a)   (b)

FIG. 9.3 Abdominal palpitation (a) for the engagement of the head,
(b) for the lie of the fetus

At each visit the legs are palpated for oedema. If there has been an excessive weight
gain the patient may complain that her wedding ring is tight. Midwives undertaking antenatal care should refer the patient to her doctor at certain invervals.
About 29 weeks is a good time for one of these examinations. Then the haemoglobin
should be checked as the blood volume is reaching its maximum. At this time, a
multiple pregnancy should be recognisable on abdominal examination. The size of
the pelvis can be assessed on vaginal examination. The nipples should be palpated to
ensure that they have become erect, ready for the baby to grasp. If the nipples are
retracted, the wearing of 'Waller's shells' (see Fig. 3.12, p. 19) can help; these shells
act by traction and initially should be worn for a short period each day, otherwise
the woman will complain of pain. By the end of one week, the patient usually
tolerates the shells for a whole day. They should be removed at night.

If the patient's blood group is Rhesus negative, a sample of blood should be sent
for testing to exclude antibody formation.

For the primigravidae, the next visit to the doctor is usually about the 34th week.
Then it is important to ensure that the vertex presents. If a breech presents, external
version can usually be performed, as the presenting part is still above the pelvic
brim. With multiparae the doctor may prefer to see the patient at the 36th week
when external version is usually possible. At these doctor's visits, any abnormal
vaginal discharge is looked for and treated. The doctor will want to see the patient
if labour fails to commence at the expected time. Postmaturity can be dangerous
especially for the baby.

Definite appointment dates for antenatal examinations should be given to the
patient, but she should be advised to see a doctor at once if bleeding occurs or if she
develops any abnormal symptoms. If the patient fails to attend, it is important to
send her a reminder or visit her at home. She may have defaulted because she felt
too ill to undertake the journey or possibly because swollen feet prevented her
from wearing outdoor shoes. It may be wise for a doctor to visit her at home or
else send her by ambulance to hospital. The home visit may be undertaken by a
Health Visitor.

Advice to the Pregnant Woman

A great deal of useful advice can be given to pregnant women, especially during a first pregnancy. It is now customary for Maternity Hospitals to hold mothercraft classes and area health authorities have done this for some time. The classes should be in the form of discussion groups, where the women have the opportunity of asking questions. Husbands may like to accompany their wives and this should be encouraged, even if it means holding evening sessions.

The classes should be planned to include the following subjects:

Diet

For fetal growth adequate *protein* is essential. First class protein occurs in meat, fish, eggs, cheese and milk. Vegetables such as peas and beans contain some second class protein. *Fats* may not be tolerated well in pregnancy. *Carbohydrates* supply energy and constitute a large part of the diet. An overweight woman should be advised to reduce her carbohydrate intake. Carbohydrates occur in potatoes, bread, sweets, etc. If the protein intake is adequate the desire for carbohydrates is reduced. The three constituents—protein, fat and carbohydrate—should supply about 2 800 calories daily.

Minerals are essential, particularly the following:

(1) *Calcium* is required, along with phosphorus, for the ossification of fetal bone. Calcium occurs in milk.

(2) *Iron*. Extra iron is needed for the increased maternal blood volume. Iron is needed for the fetal blood and storage in the large fetal liver near term. The best source of iron is in liver and red meats. The yolk of egg contains some iron, as does cocoa.

(3) *Iodine*. This is necessary for thyroid function, both maternal and fetal. Salt-water fish contain iodine, but in some countries iodine is added to common salt.

(4) *Magnesium*, *phosphorus* and various trace elements are also important, but occur along with the minerals which have been mentioned.

Sodium chloride (salt) should be used *sparingly* as it tends to cause water retention and oedema. This applies to all sodium preparations.

Vitamins are important:

Vitamin A promotes growth and increases resistance to infection. Lack of vitamin A can cause fetal abnormalities in animals (e.g. hydrocephaly in the rabbit). Vitamin A occurs in milk, butter and carrots.

Vitamin B is complex, composed of various fractions, each acting differently. Vitamin B aids both protein and carbohydrate metabolism. One constituent of vitamin B contains folic acid which is necessary to prevent megaloblastic anaemia. Vitamin B_{12} prevents pernicious anaemia, but this type of anaemia is rare until after child-bearing years. Vitamin B is necessary for the normal function of nerves and also muscles. Natural sources of vitamin B are wholemeal bread, yeast and vegetables.

Vitamin C is necessary to prevent scurvy and possibly other haemorrhages. Lack of vitamin C causes pregnant ewes to miscarry. Vitamin C helps wounds to heal. The main sources of vitamin C are citrus fruits. Potatoes contain a little under the skin. Cooking destroys vitamin C.

Vitamin D promotes the absorption of calcium and development of bone. Lack of this vitamin causes rickets. Vitamin D occurs in codliver oil and milk products.

Vitamin E is necessary to prevent miscarriages in the rat and probably also in man. Vitamin E is present in wholemeal bread, eggs and milk.

Vitamin K is essential for the formation of prothrombin. If this is reduced, bleeding occurs, e.g. epistaxis (nose-bleeding), or in the newborn baby a haemorrhagic disease. Liver is rich in vitamin K. This vitamin is also present in some green vegetables.

A daily optimum diet should include a good helping of meat, an egg, cheese, wholemeal bread, fresh fruit, vegetables and at least one pint of milk. Liver should be eaten once a week and fish at least twice. Tea and coffee should not be taken in excess because of their action on the kidneys. Alcohol is best avoided.

For many years the Government supplied vitamin A and D tablets and vitamin C as concentrated orange juice to pregnant women. They were also entitled to one pint of milk daily at a reduced price. Since April 1971 these grants have been withdrawn. Now, only if the pregnant woman has two children under the age of five years is she entitled to cheap milk.

Protein-containing foods can be expensive; however cheaper cuts of meat are often just as nutritious as the more expensive. This is also true of fish, herring giving excellent nourishment. It is foolish to insist upon women eating foods they dislike and racial habits must be respected as far as possible. A vegetarian should be instructed in the use of vegetables and dairy products; the patient's cooking facilities may be poor and advice in this respect can be helpful.

Exercise

Walking in the fresh air is best; at least one mile each day. Anything like horse-riding which jolts the pelvis, should be avoided. Swimming is unwise during the first three months, when miscarriages are common. Towards the end of pregnancy women usually will not want to swim. Cycling, avoiding hills, seems reasonable even when pregnancy is advanced.

Relaxation exercises, usually supervised by physiotherapists, are helpful both in promoting sleep and as a preparation for labour. Such exercises are generally available at Maternity Hospitals and local welfare centres.

Sleep

At least eight hours a night is important during pregnancy and during the last month the patient should rest for two hours during the afternoon.

Clothing

An expanding uplift brassière is important to support the enlarging breasts and at the same time to prevent any pressure on the developing nipples. No unnecessary bands should pass round the abdomen, therefore underskirts and dresses should hang from the shoulders. A maternity belt, again expanding, will support the pregnant abdomen and relieve some strain from the lumbar spine. Garters must be condemned because of their tendency to cause varicose veins. Shoes with a reasonably wide and low heel are advisable. High heels tend to tilt the spine forwards and cause backache.

Sexual Intercourse

This is best avoided during the first three months when miscarriages are common, and again during the last month to avoid any additional risk of infection.

Bathing

A daily bath should be taken if possible, but the water should not be excessively hot because heat to the abdomen can stimulate the uterus to contract. If a bath is not available, the vulva should be washed night and morning with soap and water. The breasts should also be washed daily. Separate flannels and towels should be used for these two areas.

Bowels

Adequate roughage in the diet should prevent constipation. If the woman normally takes aperients, the best ones to use are senna or cascara. Liquid paraffin should be avoided because it prevents ready absorption of vitamins from the intestinal tract.

Work

Many pregnant women want to continue working for financial reasons and also to enable them to receive a maternity allowance. A woman should stop work at the 28th week and not return until her baby is six weeks old. A certificate is necessary to enable her to obtain the maternity allowance. This certificate can be signed by a doctor or midwife after the 26th week of pregnancy. While at work the pregnant woman should not stand for prolonged periods. Work outside the home should be limited so that, with her home commitments, the woman is not over-tired.

Smoking

This has been shown to be associated with a 'lower than the average' baby's birth weight. This reduction in birth weight may be due to a reduction in the mother's appetite, but it is possible that nicotine is deleterious to the baby, increasing the amount of carbon monoxide received.

Preparation for labour

At mothercraft classes pregnant women, preferably accompanied by their husbands should be given a simple description of fetal growth. The signs of the onset of labour should be described, ensuring that the patient knows what to do when labour begins, i.e. how to call an ambulance for a hospital delivery or how to contact the district midwife for a home confinement. The three stages of labour should be described simply, supplemented by showing a film of a normal delivery. Simplicity is stressed, because too much detail can easily create anxiety. Inhalant analgesia apparatus should be shown and handled by the patient. In hospital the prospective parents may like to see the delivery unit.

The advantages of breast-feeding should be discussed and some possible problems.

It is important to ensure that the parents obtain suitable baby clothing and a pram, which the mother can wheel without back strain. Questions should be encouraged and answered. Pregnant women can only be invited to attend mothercraft classes. Unfortunately many of the poorer, less intelligent do not come. These can be taught, to a certain extent, during routine antenatal examination.

Unmarried Women

Pregnancy in this group is now frequent. These women require assistance, sometimes financially, as well as socially. Most Maternity Hospitals employ a medical social worker to whom the patient should be referred. Local authorities employ special health visitors for this purpose. The patient's parents should be encouraged to accept some responsibility. Midwives should ensure that unmarried women obtain adequate antenatal care.

MINOR DISORDERS OF PREGNANCY

These can worry pregnant women; often midwives can give simple advice but sometimes medical treatment is required.

Nausea

Nausea or vomiting in the early morning is fairly common during the first twelve weeks of pregnancy; the probable reason is a low blood sugar due to altered hormones. The patient should be encouraged to take a simple carbohydrate (biscuit, barley sugar or glucose) on awakening. She should rise slowly from bed.

Numerous drugs have been recommended but few, if any, do good and all are potentially dangerous at this time when the fetus is forming its essential organs. The danger of thalidomide has been well documented.

Heartburn

When the uterus rises in late pregnancy, the stomach tends to produce diminished secretions of pepsin and hydrochloric acid. The cardiac sphincter may relax and if the patient has a hiatus hernia, symptoms are aggravated. The patient should be encouraged to drink between, and not with, meals and to rest after a meal. She may benefit from sleeping with extra pillows. The consumption of fat may cause indigestion, because the liver is overtaxed during pregnancy.

If heartburn persists despite these recommendations, the doctor may prescribe dilute hydrochloric acid 0·3 ml tds before meals, mucaine, or gaviscon. Alkaline therapy is useless.

Cramp

This is common in the middle trimester when the calcium demand of the fetus is high, cramp being a form of tetany. Additional milk can help, but sometimes the doctor will prescribe calcium tablets. Low calcium can also cause excessive fetal movements. Excess phosphorus may inhibit calcium absorption and vitamin D is essential for calcium metabolism.

Cramp from pressure can only occur during the last few weeks of pregnancy after the fetal head has engaged in the pelvis.

Acroparaesthesia (carpal tunnel syndrome)

The patient complains of painful hands or fingers due to pressure on the median nerve in the carpal tunnel. Oedema is the probable cause. The pain may interfere with sleep. A reduced salt intake may help, also wearing a cock-up wrist splint during the day. After delivery, these symptoms will usually disappear.

Pelvic Arthropathy

Some relaxation of the pelvic joints during pregnancy is normal, but excessive relaxation can cause some difficulty or pain on walking. The patient will be tender over the symphysis pubis and possibly also over the sacro-iliac joints. Rest and a maternity belt may give relief. Occasionally rest in an antenatal ward is required.

Varicose Veins

A pregnant woman may worry because her leg veins become prominent or ache. Veins may also appear at the vulva or anus. They seldom thrombose. A pregnant woman should avoid standing whenever possible and sit with her legs raised. Elastic stockings tend to aggravate vulval varicose veins and are best avoided during pregnancy. The patient can be assured that her varicosities will probably diminish after delivery.

PHYSIOLOGY OF LABOUR

Labour is defined as the process by which a viable fetus (28 weeks gestation) is expelled from the uterus. The whole process is due to *retraction* of the involuntary muscles in the upper uterine segment and passive stretching of the lower uterine segment and cervix. Midwives should understand retraction. When a muscle contracts, muscle fibres shorten: with relaxation their length is restored. This action occurs in the upper uterine segment throughout pregnancy. Retraction means

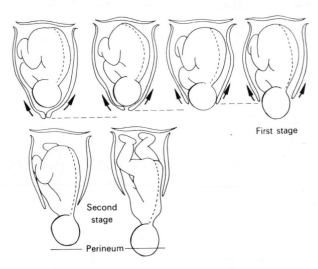

First stage

Second stage

—————— Perineum——————

FIG. 10.1 Retraction during stages of labour

that after a contraction, the muscle fibres fail to relax completely and gradually become shorter and shorter. In this way the length of the upper uterine segment diminishes. Consequently there is progressively less room for the fetus in its bag of membranes, and pressure is exerted on the lower uterine segment and cervix. The internal cervical os dilates with slight separation of the chorion from the lower segment of the uterus. The cervical canal is drawn up and disappears. Pressure on the external cervical os causes dilatation and the complete drawing up of the cervix. The period from the commencement of retraction until full dilatation of the cervix is known as the *first stage of labour*. In a primi-gravida the maximum time should not exceed 24 hours. A multiparous cervix, which has previously dilated, stretches more rapidly and the first stage should not exceed 12 hours. Frequently the time is less.

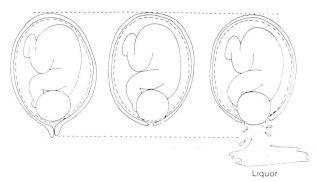

FIG. 10.2 Physiology of labour: first stage

When the cervix has dilated, the fetal membranes have no support and consequently rupture, draining liquor amnii. Continuing retraction pushes the fetus (normally head first) into the vagina which stretches, then on to the perineum

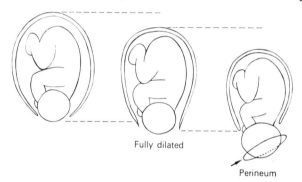

FIG. 10.3 Physiology of labour: retraction

which stretches and then the fetus is born. From the time of full dilatation of the cervix to the birth of the baby is termed the *second stage of labour*. In a primigravida this stage should not exceed 2 hours, in a multipara one hour or less.

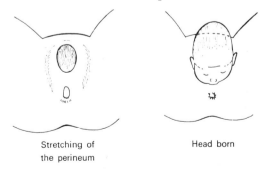

FIG. 10.4 Physiology of labour: second stage

When the lower uterine segment is drawn up the bladder will rise with it. During the 2nd stage of labour, the rectum is pushed down and the anus dilates. Because contractions and therefore retractions are intermittent, during the 2nd stage the fetal head descends and then recedes slightly, but there should be some permanent advance with each contraction. Once the fetal head begins to press on the perineum the woman desires to bear down.

During labour if the fetus lacks oxygen, its anal sphincter tends to relax and meconium is passed into the liquor amnii staining it green. Lack of oxygen can occur if the uterine contractions are excessively prolonged and frequent or if labour becomes prolonged. Early rupture of membranes causes the fetus to be directly compressed during each contraction. This can cause fetal distress.

The muscular activity of labour causes the production of extra lactic acid. This means that a patient in labour is liable to become ketosed and acetone appear in the urine. If the patient receives adequate nourishment and does not vomit, provided labour is of normal duration, ketosis should not arise.

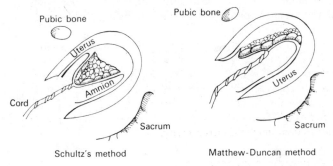

FIG. 10.5 Third stage: methods of separation

The involuntary uterine muscles are the only muscles in the body capable of retraction. The onset of retraction is probably due to a change in hormones possibly fetal adrenal changes releasing pitocin. This hormone is rendered inactive during pregnancy, probably because of progesterone. The placenta degenerates at term and probably produces less ovarian hormones. The onset of labour may also be due to the fact that the uterus can only stretch to a certain degree. Overstretching, as occurs in a multiple pregnancy or where there is excessive liquor amnii (hydramnios), tends to cause premature labour. When the fetal head engages early, pressure on the cervix can stimulate the onset of labour, especially if the circular muscles around the cervix are abnormally lax.

After the baby is born, continuing retraction of the upper uterine segment reduces the size of the placental site and causes the placenta to separate and be expelled into the vagina. When the placenta separates the whole chorionic membrane should strip off the uterine wall. In about 75 per cent of cases the central portion of the placenta separates first and the placenta is expelled fetal surface first (Shultz's separation). In the remaining 25 per cent the separation begins at a placental edge, and the placenta appears maternal surface first with the membranes trailing behind (Matthew-Duncan separation). In the latter cases, unless great care is taken, the chorionic membrane is liable to tear leaving some membrane behind in the uterus. From the birth of the baby until the placenta and membranes have been expelled, is called the *third stage of labour*. The length of this stage is independent of parity and normally should not exceed 20 minutes. Between contractions the uterus feels soft. As labour advances the contractions become more frequent, reaching one each two minutes and each lasts for a longer time. When the uterus retracts there is some ischaemia which is painful. Therefore at the onset of labour the patient is conscious of contractions. She feels some pain radiating as a rule from the back to the lower abdomen, sometimes to the upper thighs. The pain is intermittent. Dilatation of the cervix should not be painful provided the patient can relax her voluntary circular muscles around the internal os. Fear stimulates these to contract, thus interfering with the smooth stretching of the cervix and lower uterine segment and creating pain. Grantly Dick Read pointed out the importance of fear.[1]

During labour the patient's blood pressure tends to rise slightly, especially towards the end of the first stage. At this time a blood pressure of 140/90 is accepted as normal. The maternal pulse should remain below 100 per minute. The average fetal heart rate is about 140 per minute and it should not vary more than 10 beats per minute either way. Levels over 160 per minute or below 120 per minute should be regarded as dangerous.

After the third stage, retraction of the involuntary figure-of-eight shaped muscles in the upper uterine segment compress the maternal blood vessels at the placental site. Later these vessels thrombose. Continuing retraction for a few days may create 'after pains'. This is more common in multipara. Similar pain may arise if blood clot accumulates in the uterine cavity.

MECHANISM OF LABOUR

The mechanism of labour describes the passive movements which the fetus under-takes during its passage through the birth canal during labour. These movements vary with the presentation and position of the fetus.

When the vertex presents there are six possible positions i.e.

VLOA—vertex left occipito–anterior
VROA—vertex right occipito–anterior
VLOL—vertex left occipito–lateral
VROL—vertex right occipito–lateral
VLOP—vertex left occipito–posterior
VROP—vertex right occipito–posterior.

In a normal labour the occiput is anterior or lateral.

VLOA will be described. When labour begins the vertex passes through the pelvic brim, unless this has already occurred. The suboccipito-bregmatic (see Fig. 4.3) diameter (9·5 cm) passes through the right oblique diameter of the pelvic brim (12 cm). Fetal flexion is maintained and descent occurs with uterine contractions. The occiput is therefore the first part of the fetal head to reach the pelvic floor

[1] Read, G. D. (1958) *Childbirth without fear: the principles and practice of natural childbirth.* 3rd ed. Heinemann Medical Books.

muscles. The occiput is automatically rotated anteriorly to the symphysis pubis, due to the gutter shape of the pelvic floor muscles. With further descent the vertex reaches the pelvic outlet in the occipito-anterior position. Crowning occurs when the fetal head reaches the vulva.

The head is born by extension. Restitution then takes place, the fetal head

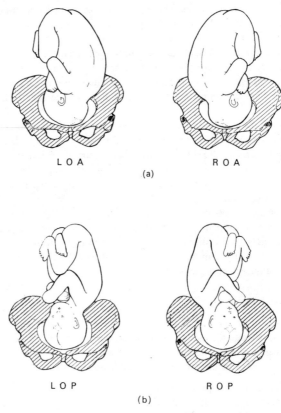

FIG. 10.6 Positions of cephalic presentation: LOA = left occipito-anterior; ROA = right occipito-anterior; ROP = right occipito-posterior; LOP = left occipito-posterior

returning to its previous flexed position and slightly oblique lie. This means the free fetal head will rotate slightly and indicates which shoulder will descend first. The next movement is that of the shoulders. They engage in the opposite oblique diameter of the pelvic brim (left oblique). The anterior shoulder descends first and, on reaching the pelvic floor, is rotated under the symphysis pubis. This rotation (known as external rotation) causes the free fetal head to turn sideways. The anterior shoulder is born first, followed by the posterior shoulder. The rest of the body is born by lateral flexion.

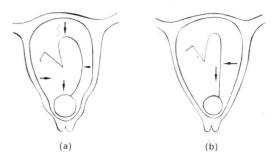

FIG. 10.7 Mechanism of labour: (a) shifting of liquor,
(b) straightening of spine

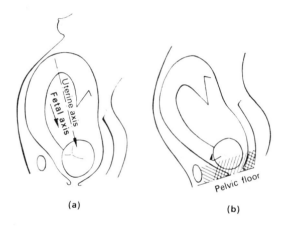

FIG. 10.8 Mechanism of labour: (a) descent, (b) rotation

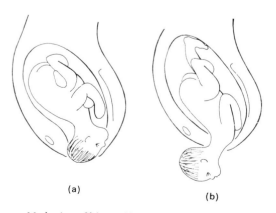

FIG. 10.9 Mechanism of labour: (a) crowning, (b) extension of the head

Asynclitism

When the fetal head engages, the anterior parietal bone usually descends in advance of the posterior parietal, i.e. the fetal head is tilted. This is known as anterior asynclitism. Occasionally the opposite occurs and this is termed posterior asynclitism.

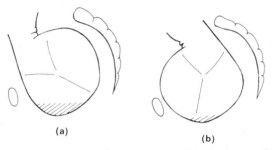

FIG. 10.10 Asynclitism: (a) anterior, (b) posterior

If the fetal membranes rupture during the first stage of labour there is direct pressure on the fetal head by the cervix. This pressure can interfere with the venous return from the fetal scalp and cause an oedematous swelling known as the *caput succedaneum*. This swelling will be over the posterior portion of the parietal bone in an occipito-anterior position and on the right side in a VLOA presentation. This swelling is superficial and therefore can cross a suture line. The swelling usually disappears within 36 hours after birth. In a difficult delayed labour the caput can become abnormally large.

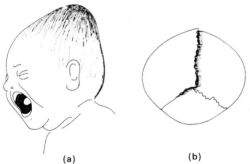

FIG. 10.11 (a) Caput succedaneum, (b) moulding

Moulding

During labour the sagittal suture allows one parietal bone to be pushed below the other and the occipital bone usually passes below the parietal bones at the lambdoidal sutures. A little moulding is advantageous as it makes the fetal head smaller. Excessive moulding, as in a difficult labour, can cause tension on the tentorium and lead to a tear and intracranial haemorrhage.

Frequently the occiput is lateral at the beginning of labour. With good contractions the fetal head will flex, engage with the suboccipito-bregmatic diameter

(9·5 cm) in the relatively wide transverse diameter of the brim (13·7 cm). The occiput should descend first so that the delivery is as described above.

MANAGEMENT OF LABOUR

When a patient thinks that labour has begun, her midwife will be called to her home if home delivery has been arranged, otherwise the patient will come to the Maternity Hospital with which she has booked. The manner in which the midwife greets the patient and relatives is important as they are usually anxious. In hospital, the patient's antenatal notes should be obtained as soon as possible.

Labour should be confirmed and a quick assessment made of the stage of labour, in case delivery is imminent. Usually the patient will be fairly early in the first stage.

To confirm labour, questions are asked as follows:

(1) Has the patient had a 'show'? This is a blood stained mucus discharge and has to be distinguished from abnormal bleeding. The mucus comes from the cervical plug in the cervical canal and the slight bleeding from the decidua above the internal os, due to separation of the chorion.

(2) When did the patient first notice uterine contractions and how often are they coming? The old term 'labour pains' should be avoided. If this term is used the patient expects pain and this will promote fright. In early normal labour there is only a degree of discomfort at the height of a contraction.

(3) Is the patient draining liquor? If so, when did this begin? Although the usual time for the membranes to rupture is at the end of the first stage of labour, the membranes may rupture early if they are abnormally fragile. The membranes may also rupture early if the circular fibres around the cervix are abnormally lax. Occasionally, involuntary micturition may be mistaken for liquor. Whilst the patient is being questioned, she is encouraged to undress and lie down on the couch or bed. When a contraction occurs the patient should relax and breathe deeply.

The midwife next confirms that everything is normal. This entails the following:

(1) Abdominal inspection and palpation, and auscultation of the fetal heart (noting the rate, rhythm and volume). In a normal labour the vertex may have engaged deeply in the pelvis out of abdominal reach.

(2) Examination of the patient's general condition, by taking her blood pressure, pulse and temperature.

The midwife will inspect the vulva, wearing an efficient mask covering her mouth and nose in order to prevent droplet infection. She will look for evidence of a show (inspection of the sanitary pad the patient is wearing is better). The midwife will note if liquor is draining. Vernix distinguishes liquor from urine. If the patient is asked to bear down, usually liquor if draining, can be seen to come from the vagina.

If labour has obviously become established, it is wise to ascertain the degree of cervical dilatation. The simplest method and the least disturbing to the patient is by a rectal examination.

Rectal Examination

Provided the midwife is right handed, the patient should turn onto her left side and flex her thighs and legs. After explaining the procedure, the midwife inserts her index finger (covered with a well lubricated finger stall) into the patient's anus.

The midwife will feel the hard smooth fetal head and can determine whether it is above or below the level of the ischial spines. The cervix is palpated through the anterior rectal wall, and the cervical os is examined. The size of the cervical opening can be determined by pressing gently against the fetal head. In early labour the os may only admit one finger. After this it should be possible to assess whether the cervix is a quarter, a third, a half or even threequarters dilated. The last portion of the cervix to disappear is the anterior rim. In a normal labour the cervix should feel soft and easily dilatable. The thickness of the cervix should be noted. Membranes may be felt bulging through the os, especially when a contraction occurs. If the

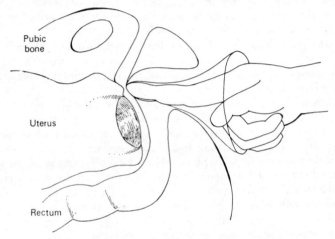

FIG. 10.12 Rectal examination

membranes have already ruptured, the soft caput may be felt. When the examination has been completed, the midwife withdraws her finger, disposes of the finger-stall and swabs the perineum and anus from before backwards with an antiseptic solution, e.g. hibitane. The midwife should then wash her hands thoroughly. The rectum is never sterile, consequently organisms may be withdrawn with the fingerstall.

An alternative and more accurate method of confirming the presenting part and state of the cervix is by a vaginal examination. This is more disturbing to the patient and risks the introduction of infection, especially after the membranes have rup-tured. With aseptic and antiseptic precautions a midwife should not hesitate to perform a vaginal exmination if she considers one to be a necessity. This method may be preferable (less painful) to a rectal examination if the patient has haemor-rhoids.

Vaginal Examination

The midwife, wearing an adequate mask, must scrub her hands carefully and put on a sterile glove. The patient should be in the dorsal position with thighs flexed and her feet on the couch or bed. The midwife will be on the patient's right side. The vulval area is swabbed with a suitable antiseptic lotion, e.g. hibitane. The labia are

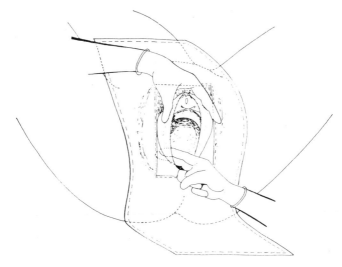

FIG. 10.13 Vaginal examination

separated with two fingers of the midwife's left hand and the midwife inserts two fingers of the gloved hand, lubricated with hibitane cream, into the vagina and feels the presenting part, the degree of cervical dilatation, sometimes described in cm, and the softness and thickness of the cervix. If the membranes have ruptured,

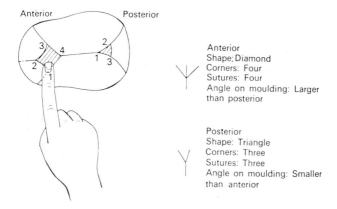

Anterior
Shape; Diamond
Corners: Four
Sutures: Four
Angle on moulding: Larger
than posterior

Posterior
Shape: Triangle
Corners: Three
Sutures: Three
Angle on moulding: Smaller
than anterior

FIG. 10.14 Palpation and recognition of fontanelles

the midwife should be able to feel the sagittal suture, and in a normal labour, the posterior fontanelle lying anterior to the median line. The fetal position can be confirmed by feeling a fetal ear. The smooth part of the external auricle faces the occiput, the irregular anterior opening being in front. To feel an ear the examining fingers may have to be passed quite high up into the vagina. When a vaginal examination is being done the patient can inhale an analgesic gas, e.g. nitrous oxide

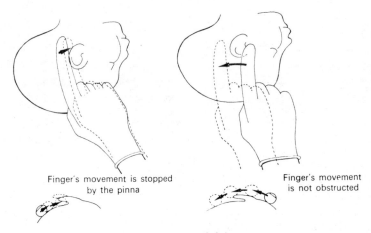

Finger's movement is stopped
by the pinna

Finger's movement
is not obstructed

FIG. 10.15 How to feel the ear

and oxygen or penthrane to minimise discomfort. In a normal labour the intact
membranes should feel globular and the cervix should be closely applied to the
fetal head.

After confirming that the patient is in labour and that delivery is not imminent,
the patient is prepared as follows:

(1) The patient empties her bladder. A mid-stream specimen of urine should be
tested for protein, glucose, pus and acetone. A trace of protein is quite common
during labour.

(2) Hair is shaved from the vulva and mons pubis using a sharp razor blade with
soap and water. Without hair it is easier to disinfect the region.

(3) The lower bowel is emptied. Various types of suppository (e.g. beogex) have
been tried but are not so effective as an enema. This should be given through a
rubber tube and funnel using soft soap and warm water. Unless the lower bowel is
empty, faeces can occupy valuable space in the pelvis and during the second stage of
labour defaecation will occur. This is naturally distressing to the patient and also
increases the risk of infection to both mother and baby.

(4) The patient is given a warm bath. This refreshes her and heat to the abdomen
stimulates the uterus to contract.

Observation during the preparatory stage, e.g. the frequency and strength of the
uterine contractions and the degree of cervical dilatation enables an experienced
midwife to judge approximately how long labour will last.

MANAGEMENT OF THE FIRST STAGE OF LABOUR

A simple sedative can relieve an anxious patient. Chloral hydrate in the form of
Welldorm tablets (1200 mg) orally is commonly used or Doriden (glutethemide)
0·25 mg. If it is daytime the patient in a normal labour can remain up and about,
keeping herself occupied. She is encouraged to relax, breathing deeply during a
contraction. Her mind should be occupied by reading, knitting or listening to the
radio. The presence of her husband can help enormously. Otherwise a midwife

should be in constant attendance or readily available, the patient having facilities (usually in hospital by a bedside bell) to call for attention.

Important nursing duties include:

(1) Ensuring that the patient empties her bladder frequently, at least 3 hourly. In a normal labour this is usually spontaneous, especially if the patient is allowed to get out of bed.

(2) *Feeding.* Suitable nourishment is necessary to prevent ketosis. In labour, however, patients tend to vomit and their stomachs empty slowly; also the patient may require an anaesthetic before labour is complete. Food should therefore be sieved. Fluids such as water and tea are necessary. Glucose drinks can cause fatal irritation if they reach the lungs and therefore should be avoided.

(3) Regular observation of the progress of labour is necessary to ensure that everything is normal. The fetal heart should be counted and recorded about every 2 hours (but not if this involves wakening a sleeping patient). The mother's pulse should be taken at the same time and the strength and frequency of the uterine contractions recorded. About every 4 hours the patient's blood pressure and temperature should be recorded.

(4) *The relief of pain.* With modern drugs a midwife should not allow a patient to become distressed with pain during labour. However, a relaxed patient, provided labour is normal, may not wish to have analgesics (pain relieving drugs) and none should be forced on her. All analgesics are potentially dangerous to the fetus, especially if the baby is born with a low birth weight. Midwives can use the following drugs if they have been instructed in their use:

(a) *Pethidine.* This depresses the fetal respiratory centre and should not be given within 4 hours of the expected time of delivery. If pethidine is given before labour is truly established, the uterine contractions may diminish or even cease and labour be prolonged. Once pethidine has been given, the patient should remain in bed. She will usually sleep for a few hours possibly arousing with contractions. Obstetricians have differing opinions regarding optimum dosage of pethidine and the midwife will learn this at her midwifery training hospital. Some patients are sensitive to pethidine and vomit. When this is known a more expensive drug, fortral, can be given.

(b) *Inhalation analgesia.* For many years midwives have been encouraged to give a mixture of nitrous oxide and air in approved machines to patients in labour. This reduced the oxygen supply to the fetus and the method is now obsolete. A 50 per cent mixture of nitrous oxide and oxygen can now be used in approved machines. This is safer for the fetus but is not such a satisfactory analgesic. Trilene can be given by midwives in a standard machine but there is some evidence that this is dangerous if the patient has already had pethidine. Recently penthrane has been approved by the Central Midwives Board for use in a fixed dose of 0·35 per cent. The best time to begin an inhalant analgesic is towards the end of the first stage of labour. At this time a patient, especially a multipara, may tend to 'bear down' onto an undilated cervix. If she inhales the analgesic during contractions she is unable to push.

The patient may continue to use the inhalant analgesic during the second stage of labour. If she feels like 'bearing down' she should inhale as soon as a contraction begins, taking four deep breaths, then, keeping the mask on her face, she can push.

She can take two further breaths and push again, and continue until her uterus relaxes. During the actual delivery of the fetal head the patient should inhale continuously and not push.

The pain threshold of patients varies immensely. Pressure of the fetal head on the perineum can be painful, especially in a first delivery. Spraying the posterior fourchette and perineum with xylocaine relieves pain.

During the first stage of labour, when the patient is in bed she should avoid the dorsal position, and lie on her side, preferably on the opposite one to the fetal back. Lying on her back can cause pressure on the inferior vena cava by the uterus, making the patient feel faint and interfering with the placental blood supply to the fetus. When the membranes rupture the midwife must note the quantity and colour of the liquor and check the fetal heart sounds.

SECOND STAGE

In a normal labour it is usually obvious when the second stage of labour has been reached. This is the normal time for the membranes to rupture. The anus dilates. Soon the fetal head becomes visible during a contraction. With each contraction the fetal head descends but recedes slightly when the uterus relaxes. This to and fro motion allows the vagina to stretch gradually and later the perineum. During the second stage of labour the patient instinctively tends to 'bear down' or push, but sometimes not until the fetal head has reached the perineum.

During the second stage of labour the midwife should not leave her patient. The midwife must ensure that a cot is being heated for the baby and a sterile delivery pack is at hand. This should not be opened sooner than necessary.

During the second stage the patient can choose her most comfortable position. If she wishes she can use an inhalant analgesic. She may 'push' if she desires to, but it is useless to enforce this. The fetal heart and maternal pulse should be checked frequently, at least every ten minutes.

As soon as the fetal head reaches the perineum the midwife wearing an efficient

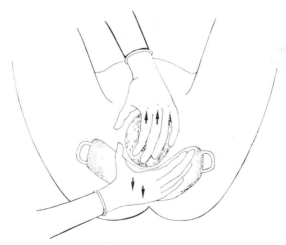

FIG. 10.16 Guarding the perineum

mask, must open the sterile delivery pack, and give herself plenty of time to 'scrub up' and put on sterile gloves. The optimum position for delivery is the left lateral. In this position the midwife can observe the perineum and control the exit of the fetal head and shoulders. The perineum and vulva should be disinfected using an efficient antiseptic lotion, e.g. hibitane. A gamgee dressing can be held over the anus to prevent contamination but no pressure should be exerted. It is important to allow the fetal head to advance naturally until it is crowned (biparietal diameters free at the vulva). Thereafter a slow exit is important to avoid any perineal laceration. The midwife should hold the fetal head with her right hand grasping the parietal bones, thumb on one side and fingers on the other. Between contractions the midwife can extend the fetal head gently. After the fetal head has been born the

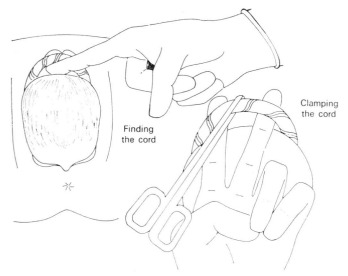

Clamping
the cord

Finding
the cord

FIG. 10.17 Cord round the baby's neck

midwife should feel to make sure that the umbilical cord is not around the fetal neck. If the cord is there, the cord must be divided between Spencer Well's forceps and delivery hastened; otherwise the baby will become asphyxiated. Normally no cord will be felt. Before the uterus contracts again the midwife has time to wipe the baby's eyelids with swabs moistened with sterile water using one separate sterile swab for each eyelid. The fetal head will turn sideways when the shoulders rotate on the pelvic floor (external rotation); with the next contraction the anterior shoulder should emerge under the symphysis pubis and be born. The midwife can help by grasping the head biparietally using both hands, one on each side and easing the head gently backwards. Excess traction is dangerous, straining the fetal neck. Once the anterior shoulder has been born the posterior shoulder follows, but the midwife can help by bringing the fetal head forwards towards the maternal abdomen. The fetal body will follow by lateral flexion. It is important that the shoulders are born in the antero-posterior (widest) diameter of the outlet to prevent tearing of the perineum. With the birth of the baby some liquor is usually expelled and there may be slight bleeding. Sometimes there is a slight delay between the birth of the head and shoulders. The midwife can ascertain that the fetal circulation remains satisfactory by pressing the fetal scalp, and on releasing her finger the blanched area will quickly become pink. If there is any delay, with the next contraction the patient should be encouraged to push down. Midwives should refrain from touching the axillae or shoulders.

After the baby has been born the cord vessels usually continue to pulsate for a few minutes enabling the baby to receive additional blood; more may be received if the baby lies lower than the placental site. Usually the baby is placed over the

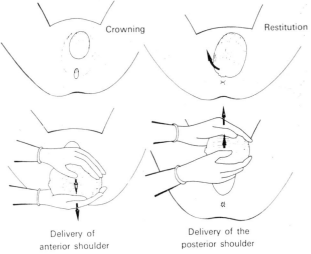

Crowning

Restitution

Delivery of
anterior shoulder

Delivery of the
posterior shoulder

FIG. 10.18 Management of labour: second stage

mother's left leg, with the baby's head lower than its body. Lowering the head encourages liquor and mucus to drain from the baby's pharynx, but before the baby breathes it is wise to extract any mucus, using a sterile mucus catheter. The baby's first breath is an inspiration. The baby may not breathe or cry until the placental circulation has ceased, but should be pink and of good muscular tone. The time of delivery should be noted.

When the cord has ceased to pulsate, the cord should be securely clamped and divided with sterile scissors about 5 cm from the baby's umbilicus. The maternal end of the cord should be placed in a sterile receiver. After showing a healthy baby to its mother, the baby wrapped in a warm towel and blankets, should be placed on its right side in the warm cot from which any electric blanket or hot water bottle has been removed. If placed on its left side the baby's heart may prevent full expansion of the left lung.

THIRD STAGE

As soon as the midwife is satisfied that the baby is breathing well and of good colour, she should concentrate upon the third stage. The mother will be encouraged to turn onto her back and the cord should be straightened. Any necessary cord

blood samples will be collected into appropriate tubes. It is customary to clamp
the maternal end of the cord at the same time as the fetal end, but, if the cord has
ceased to pulsate, there should be little bleeding from the maternal side.

Whilst awaiting placental separation, the midwife should keep one hand on the
uterine fundus and watch for any vaginal bleeding. Uterine contractions will be
felt and their frequency determines the probable length of the third stage. When the
placenta has separated the uterine fundus will rise, become more mobile and hard
and there is usually slight vaginal bleeding. A useful test for placental separation is
to press gently above the symphysis pubis and upwards. If the placenta is free the

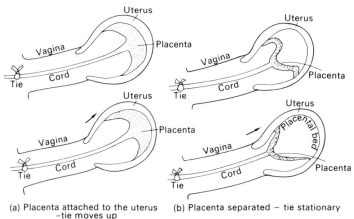

(a) Placenta attached to the uterus
    –tie moves up

(b) Placenta separated – tie stationary

FIG. 10.19 Test for separation of the placenta

cord will not change, but if the placenta is still attached to the uterine wall the cord
will recede towards the vagina. The placenta after separation is expelled into the
vagina, from there the mother may be able to push it out, but sometimes the midwife will require to use gentle uterine pressure. No bleeding should occur during
the third stage until the placenta separates. The placenta should not be allowed to
tumble out because the membranes may tear. The midwife should receive the
placenta in her hands and ease the membranes out, if necessary twisting them to add
strength. If the membranes tear some will be left within the uterus and encourage
later infection. The membranes are more liable to tear if the placenta appears
maternal surface first (Matthew–Duncan separation). With the separation and
delivery of the placenta there is some bleeding. The amount varies with the size
of the placenta but usually will not exceed 300 ml. Afterwards the bleeding should
cease and the uterus remain well contracted. After swabbing the vulval area, the
midwife should inspect the labia, vagina and perineum in case any laceration has
occurred. All soiled linen should be removed and the patient made comfortable.
Her blood pressure, pulse rate and temperature should be recorded.

The placenta and membranes must be examined carefully to make sure they are
complete. The opening in the membranes will show the position of the placental
site, whether in the upper uterine segment or lower. The placenta is weighed and
any infarcts or abnormal calcification noted. The cord length is recorded and the

number of cord vessels; normally there are 2 arteries and 1 vein. The type of cord insertion should be recorded. The blood loss is measured. This blood has in the past been thrown away; now some drug firms are anxious to collect the blood for the manufacture of products such as γ globulin. After the midwife is sure that everything is normal she should give the mother a hot drink.

During the third stage the midwife should be able to observe the baby and it is wise to check that there has been no bleeding from the cord; the clamp might slip or cut through a thick cord. The loss of 1 oz (30 ml) of blood is comparable to the loss of one pint in an adult.

A midwife must remain with her patient for at least one hour after delivery. This gives her time to deal with the baby. Its weight and length should be recorded. The midwife should look for any abnormality of the mouth, limbs, spine, anus and external genitalia. The baby's face and head should be washed but most paediatricians consider it wise to leave the body coated with vernix. This protects the skin from infection. The umbilical cord should be dressed and the baby clothed. The baby's temperature should be recorded using a rectal thermometer. In hospital an identification tape should be attached to the baby recording the name, weight and time of birth.

Before leaving the midwife must check that the mother's uterus is well contracted and that there is no bleeding. It is wise to recheck the pulse rate and blood pressure. In hospital the mother should not be moved from the delivery unit within one hour.

For many years midwives have given 2 ergot tablets after delivery. They contain all three ergot alkaloids both fast and slow acting: time is required for absorption but the uterus will be stimulated to contract for several hours. If, however, the midwife feels the uterus is not well contracted after the third stage, she can inject either 0·5 mg ergometrine intramuscularly (IM) or the more potent (and more expensive) syntometrine which contains 5 units synthetic pitocin as well as 0·5 mg ergometrine. Their action is much more rapid than can be expected from tablets, but the effect wears off quickly.

A normal delivery has been described in some detail. Unfortunately at this present age of speed, there is a tendency to encourage midwives to hasten both the second and third stages of labour. The perineum can be incised (episiotomy) but this is seldom necessary in a normal labour. Some obstetricians advocate an episiotomy to prevent future prolapse. A midwife must be taught how to perform an

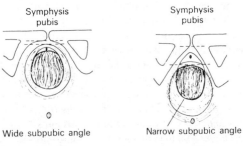

Fig. 10.20 Diagram to show how a narrow subpubic angle wastes available space and may necessitate an episiotomy

episiotomy in an emergency, but should realise an episiotomy can be painful at the time and during the early puerperium and extra bleeding will occur. The usual type of episiotomy is a medio-lateral incision involving the levator ani. Once muscle has been cut, future functions may alter. Dysparunia may result. At a

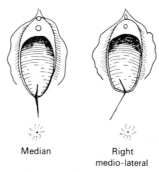

Median   Right medio-lateral

FIG. 10.21 Episiotomies

future delivery the scarred tissue is incapable of stretching normally and in most cases another episiotomy will be required. Because of unsatisfactory results from a medio-lateral episiotomy, many obstetricians now favour a median one. Should

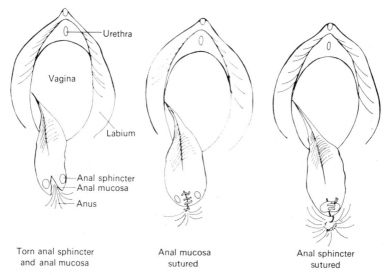

Torn anal sphincter and anal mucosa   Anal mucosa sutured   Anal sphincter sutured

FIG. 10.22 Third degree tear

this incision extend, the anal sphincter is easily involved (third degree tear). Another possible incision is J-shaped but this can be difficult to suture.

Midwives must know how to perform an episiotomy in an emergency to prevent a severe perineal tear or prolonged pressure of a small fetal head on the perineum. An undiagnosed breech presentation necessitates an episiotomy unless the perineum is lax. Recently the Central Midwives Board has suggested that midwives should inject 2 ml lignocaine before performing an episiotomy in order to reduce the pain of the incision. This local anaesthetic takes up to 5 minutes to give anaesthesia and the actual injection causes some discomfort. If midwives only perform an episiotomy as an emergency, they will seldom if ever have time to give an effective local anaesthetic.

Recently midwives have been encouraged to hasten the third stage of labour and minimise blood loss by injecting 1 ml syntometrine intramuscularly (IM) (0·5 mg ergometrine and 5 units synthetic pictocin) with the crowning of the fetal head or delivery of the anterior shoulder. This timing is unfortunate, coinciding with the time when the midwife should be concentrating on the actual delivery. If the

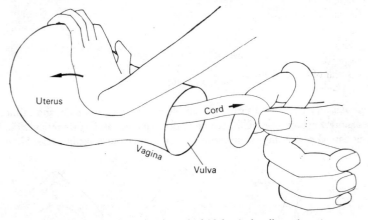

FIG. 10.23 Brandt–Andrew's method (abdominal wall not drawn)

injection is given too early a constriction ring may prevent easy delivery of the shoulders and head. An undiagnosed twin might die in utero from asphyxia.

There is no logical reason for giving syntometrine at this stage. Midwives should be supplied with syntometrine and not hesitate to give it should any abnormal bleeding occur during the third stage or after. Later administration does not increase the incidence of a constriction ring. Before giving the injection the midwife should have had time to deal with the baby and palpate the uterus, excluding a twin. Once syntometrine has been given the midwife should concentrate on the uterus and recognise when placental separation occurs so that there is no delay in its expulsion. Oxytoxic drugs such as syntometrine may raise the mother's blood pressure if she has toxaemia.

Brandt–Andrew's method of delivering the placenta by cord traction has been recommended. The uterus must be well contracted and a hand placed on the lower uterine segment. Unless the placenta has separated the cord may break. Sometimes the uterus will invert creating serious shock but more often some placental tissue or membrane is left within the uterus. Secondary haemorrhage or infection may occur. The optimal blood loss at delivery is not known. Some blood returns to the maternal circulation when the uterus retracts after the third stage. The larger the placental site the more blood loss can be expected.

This interference with the third stage in a physiological event merits serious reconsideration. Why hurry a normal event?

A midwife is trained to deal with a normal delivery and she should strive to achieve this, never interfering with nature without serious thought. Midwives must recognise any complication early and obtain medical aid promptly:

(1) Any presentation other than a vertex.

(2) A high fetal head in a primigravida.

(3) Early rupture of membranes without labour contractions.

(4) Labour commencing before 36 weeks gestation.

(5) Fetal or maternal distress.

(6) Prolongation of any stage of labour.

(7) Any bleeding during the third stage of labour.

(8) Postpartum haemorrhage (loss exceeding 600 ml) or the mother showing signs of shock.

(9) Suspected incomplete placenta.

(10) Any tear of the genital tract or perineum.

(11) Fetal asphyxia or abnormality.

11   CARE OF THE NEWBORN BABY

This is a large subject about which many excellent books have been written. Only the essential care by a midwife will be described.

If labour occurs before 36 weeks gestation, the delivery should be in hospital with a doctor in attendance. If a 'small for dates' (dysmature) infant is suspected the midwife must seek medical aid.

With a normal delivery and a healthy mother, the baby should breathe and cry immediately the cord is divided, but it is important to clear mucus from the air passages with a sterile mucus catheter before the first inspiration. The baby should be kept warm and its temperature checked, but because a newborn baby's skin is so delicate and its cry of distress may not be heeded, no hot water bottles (or electric blanket) must be left inside the cot, warm blankets are adequate.

Asphyxia Neonatorum

Asphyxia cannot always be anticipated but may occur in prolonged labour, in abnormal and instrumental deliveries and as a result of placental insufficiency. The severity varies and is best assessed by use of the Apgar scoring system, if possible at one and five minutes after birth. Up to 2 points are scored for each sign.

Apgar Score, to be read at one minute after birth or later

Sign	Score		
	0	1	2
Heart rate	Absent	Below 100	Over 100
Respiration	Absent	Weak cry	Good cry
Tone	None	Some flexion of extremities	Active movement
Response to catheter insertion into the nose	Nil	Grimace	Cough or sneeze
Colour	Pale or blue	Body pink, extremities blue	Pink all over

In mild cases the baby retains its muscle tone and its reflexes but is cyanosed and fails to breathe at once. Usually the baby will respond to simple aspiration of mucus from the pharynx, oxygen by face mask can then be given. Generally the baby responds quickly and the outlook is good. If pethidine has been given within 4 hours of birth, the antidote lethidrone can be injected by a doctor, 0·25–1 mg.

In severe cases (Apgar score 3 or below) the baby is shocked and in urgent need of oxygen. A midwife rarely encounters this unaided if she has recognised fetal distress during labour and obtained medical aid. Such a baby is pale and limp, the heart may be beating feebly and reflexes are poor or absent. Cardiac massage is necessary only when the circulation stops and must be sufficiently forceful to produce palpable pulsation in the femoral vessels. A doctor must be called urgently as intubation of the larynx may be necessary, also administration of sodium bicarbonate intravenously to combat acidosis. Aspiration of mucus and administration of oxygen by face mask should be carried out whilst awaiting medical assistance.

Examination of the Baby

The midwife must examine every baby thoroughly for any obvious deformity, e.g. mouth, limbs and spine. The umbilical cord should be checked for three vessels and must be watched for bleeding. Various methods of treatment for the cord have been advocated and the midwife will learn one at her training hospital.

Later Care

(1) *Temperature.* The rectal temperature is usually recorded daily. It should be between 36–37°C.

(2) *Weight.* All new-born babies lose weight initially (due to the passage of urine and meconium and loss of fluid through the skin and by respiration), but normally not more than 8 per cent birth weight. After the 3rd day the weight should rise by 32–64 ml per kg daily and the birth weight should be regained within 2 weeks. It is customary to weigh a baby shortly after birth, on the 3rd day and afterwards on alternate days if all is progressing satisfactorily.

(3) *Colour.* Normally the colour is pink, although for some hours the extremities may remain slightly blue.

Abnormal colouration:

(a) *Pallor.* This could mean that bleeding is taking place, either from the cord or internally. It may also indicate an infection.

(b) *Jaundice.* If this appears within 36 hours of birth the cause is usually Rhesus immunisation or an ABO blood incompatibility. Such complications should have been detected antenatally. Jaundice appearing after 36 hours is usually physiological due to the breakdown of the extra fetal cells. This jaundice should disappear by the 5th day. Continuing jaundice can be due to infection arising, as a rule from the umbilicus. There are other rare causes. If the bilirubin level rises above 15 mg per 100 ml (250 S.I. units), phototherapy is indicated, protecting the baby's eyes. If the bilirubin should reach 25 mg per 100 ml (425 S.I. units) an exchange blood transfusion becomes necessary.

(c) *Cyanosis.* Inhalation of meconium or inhaled vomit may cause cyanosis. A baby with a congenital heart deformity may also show cyanosis especially on crying.

(4) *General Condition.* During the first week a baby should sleep most of the time only awakening when hungry. The cry should be of a normal pitch (a high pitched cry denotes a possible cerebral injury or meningitis). The Moro sign should be present (Fig. 11.1).

(5) *Stools.* At first the stools are brownish green, i.e. meconium. They change to a yellow colour after a few days. After this any loose offensive stools, especially

if they contain mucus or blood denote infection. Blood in the stool may give it a tarry appearance. An overfed baby may have bulky frequent stools. An underfed baby tends to pass small frequent hard, sometimes green, stools.

(6) The umbilical cord usually separates by a process of dry gangrene on the 4th or 5th day. Delayed separation may be due to infection. The cord should never be offensive. Redness around the umbilicus means infection. Careful treatment of the cord in order to prevent infection is vital. Various techniques are employed.

(7) *Feeding*. Human milk is the best for a human baby. The early colostrum contains easily digested protein and fat and also lysozymes besides other substances, which

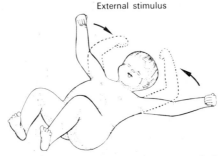

External stimulus

FIG. 11.1. Moro reflex. A normal baby reacts to any external stimulus, such as shaking the cot, by moving limbs as depicted in the diagram.

protect the baby against infection. The baby wants to feed frequently at first, although there is little breast milk for the first few days. Mature human milk is only formed after a few weeks. The baby should be encouraged to suck when awake and apparently hungry. During the day the interval between feeds should not exceed 4 hours. Occasionally some medical condition of the mother, e.g. pulmonary tuberculosis makes breast feeding inadvisable. In some rare cases the maternal nipples are hopelessly inverted. Sometimes the mother does not wish to breast feed her baby. In these cases artificial feeding with a cow's milk preparation becomes necessary.

Artificial Feeding

Numerous artificial foods are marketed. It probably matters little which product is used. All except 'humanised' preparations exaggerate the tendency to hypocalcaemia in the new-born. It is very essential that midwives know the fluid and calorie requirements of a baby during the first two weeks of life. Fluid is essential and later calories. Five per cent dextrose can be given during the first 24 hours, the amount varying with the individual baby. Thereafter artificial cow's milk can be given each 30 ml containing 20 calories. The baby usually requires about ½ oz per lb body weight (32 ml per kg) initially and by gradual increments will require 2½ oz per lb birth weight (160 ml per kg) by the end of one week. In hospital nowadays artificial feeds are usually prepared in a central milk unit. For home confinements the midwife must ensure that the feeds are prepared and kept sterile. Before the milk is given to the baby it should be warmed to a temperature of 37·2°C (99°F). The teats can be disinfected by immersion in Milton and the bottles should be boiled.

(8) *Infection.* A newborn baby has little resistance to infection. The usual sites are the skin, eyes, umbilicus, lungs and intestinal tract. The midwife can reduce the incidence of infection by carefully washing her hands between handling different babies. Sterile equipment is essential. Vernix which covers the skin at birth is protective and should not be removed. Early washing should be of the face and skin folds only. In hospital an infected baby must be isolated, preferably with the mother.

Ophthalmia Neonatorum

By definition this means a purulent discharge from the eye within 21 days of birth. The doctor must notify this to the Area Health Officer. The reason is to prevent blindness by early diagnosis and treatment. In the old days the causal organism was the gonococcus, now staphylococci are more common.

The midwife must obtain medical aid whenever she notices a discharge from a baby's eye.

Low weight babies 'weighing 2500 g or less at birth' require extra care in special premature baby units, and midwives who intend to look after such babies will require special training.

Before the baby leaves hospital it is important that the midwife has taught the mother how to care for her baby. Such education is equally important in home deliveries.

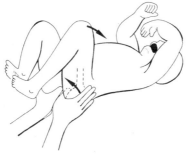

Fig. 11.2. Barlow's test for dislocation of the hips is performed by abducting the hips to ensure there is no hip click

The doctor will have examined the baby thoroughly for any obvious abnormality. All midwives should be able to carry out Barlow's test for detection of hip dislocation.

Rarely (1 in 20 000) babies are born without normal enzymes. Phenylketonuria, if it occurs, can be detected in a baby's urine or blood within the first week of life. 5 ml acidified urine is added to a few drops of 5–10 per cent aqueous solution of ferric chloride. If the urine lacks phenylalanine a green colour will develop within a few minutes. The blood test 'Guthrie' is more sensitive and the blood sample can be tested in laboratories for additional amino-acid defects. If phenylketonuria is detected early, permanent brain damage can be prevented by giving special diet. Midwives should be taught about the urine test and how to obtain a blood sample by heel prick.

Any baby who has required resuscitation at birth or shown any abnormal signs early in life must be 'followed up' by a paediatrician, preferably at the hospital where the child was born. Only there are full records available.

A normal baby will be followed up at home by a Health Visitor. If the baby had a low birth weight, specially trained health visitors will visit the baby after the baby goes home. Arrangements for the follow up care are made through the midwives' supervisor of the Area Health Authority.

This is the period following delivery during which the genital organs return approximately to their pre-pregnant condition. The uterus remains slightly larger than in a nullipara and the external cervical os has a slight lateral slit in place of the circular opening (provided the delivery has been per vaginam).

The uterus should diminish in size and resume its normal anteverted, anteflexed position in the pelvis. The initial shrinkage is by continuing retraction of the involuntary muscles. Later, superfluous muscle and blood vessels are absorbed by autolysis. The uterine ligaments shrink and regain their tone. During autolysis protein metabolites reach the blood and are excreted in the urine. The whole

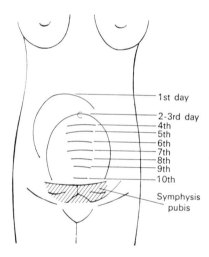

FIG. 12.1 Uterine involution in the puerperium

process is termed involution. Involution is rapid during the first two weeks and can be checked by measuring the height of the uterine fundus above the symphysis pubis, after the bladder has been emptied. The average height after delivery is 12·5 cm. This normally diminishes 1·25 cm daily so that the fundus returns to the pelvis by the 10th day. Involution is slower in a multipara than a primipara. It is slow if the mother fails to breast feed. Obviously, an excessively large uterus (e.g. after twins or hydramnios) takes longer than normal to return to the pelvis, even if shrinkage is at the rate of 1·25 cm daily. Infection or retained products such as placental tissue, membrane, blood clot or lochia slow down the process of involution. A fibroid uterus will remain permanently large.

Lochia

This is the uterine discharge following delivery. For 48 hours lochia consists mainly of blood and is bright red. The quantity should not be excessive, i.e. two sanitary pads should hold the lochia, but the pads require to be changed every 3 hours during the day. The lochia remains red for 3–4 days and then becomes brown, and by the end of two weeks is scanty and yellow. In addition to blood, lochia contains the decidual cells which are shed from the uterine wall. If the uterus becomes infected, the lochia will be offensive.

To aid involution the mother should breast feed. Drainage of lochia should be encouraged by posture, i.e. by allowing the patient out of bed or when in bed to sit upright or be in the prone position. This latter position brings the cervix away from the symphysis pubis and promotes better drainage. Infection must be prevented (see below).

Management of the puerperium includes the following:

(1) Care of the general health of the mother.
(2) Maintenace of uterine asepsis.
(3) Promotion of breast feeding (if possible).
(4) Education of the mother in the management of her baby.

GENERAL HEALTH OF THE MOTHER

After delivery a mother wants to sleep. Unfortunately, the baby may wish to feed during the night and therefore the mother should be allowed some time to sleep during the day as well. Excitement may make her wakeful at first. In this case a doctor may prescribe Welldorm 1200 mg orally. 'After pains' or a painful perineum may necessitate paracetamol. Aspirin, because it contains salicylate, should be avoided if the mother is breast feeding. Drugs pass via the breast milk to the baby. Salicylates combine with albumin and in the early days of life the baby requires albumin to combine with bilirubin arising from the breakdown of fetal blood cells; otherwise the baby may become jaundiced.

Diet is just as important as during pregnancy. The mother's temperature occasionally rises immediately after delivery (stress–strain reaction) but this is unusual after a completely normal labour. After this the temperature should remain normal. On the 3rd or 4th day when milk comes in, engorgement of the breasts may occur and the temperature may rise. The pulse rate should remain normal. A raised pulse rate and temperature denote infection.

Because of increased metabolites due to uterine autolysis there is a diuresis and the mother needs to micturate frequently. She may however find micturition difficult, due to decreased intra-abdominal pressure, reduction of bladder muscular tone, or fear of pain if there has been any vaginal or perineal tear. She may find a bed pan difficult to use. Early ambulation can help.

If a patient has a full bladder and is unable to micturate medical aid must be called. The doctor will probably prescribe an injection of ubretid. Catheterisation is only done if all else fails. It is impossible to introduce a catheter into the bladder without risk of urinary infection. A midwife must never catheterise a patient without real reason. Constipation is common because of the lax abdominal muscles. An aperient on the 2nd evening is often necessary, e.g. sennakot.

Postnatal Exercises

Exercises for the lower limbs are important to prevent puerperal thrombosis. Deep breathing exercises are especially important if the patient has had a general anaesthetic. Exercises for the pelvic floor muscles are vital if the muscles are to

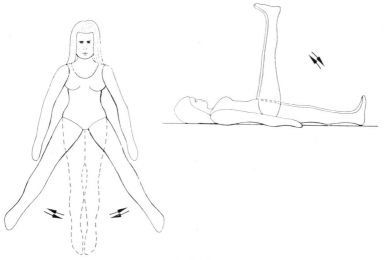

FIG. 12.2 Perineal exercises

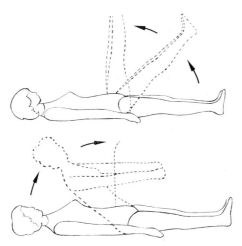

FIG. 12.3 Exercises for abdominal muscles

regain their tone. Abdominal exercises should also be done. All exercises are best done under the supervision of trained physiotherapists. If the delivery has been at home the midwife will usually have to be responsible for seeing that exercises are done.

MAINTENANCE OF UTERINE ASEPSIS

All foci of infection e.g. dental caries should have been dealt with, as far as possible, during the antenatal period. After the birth, it is important that the complete placenta and all membranes are expelled. The uterus should not be allowed to fill up with blood. Lochia should drain freely. Autogenous infection by the patient herself should be avoided, e.g. disposable paper handkerchiefs should be used. The patient must be taught to wash her hands well before touching the vulva. Sanitary pads must be sterile. After defaecation the perineum must be swabbed from before backwards. If the patient is allowed to get up, cross infection from lavatory seats must be prevented. Any nurse swabbing the vulva or treating sutures must wear a gown, mask and sterile gloves to prevent cross-infection. In hospital, wards should not be overcrowded. Any patient with infection should be isolated. Only healthy visitors should be permitted. Floors should be damp dusted or oiled. No midwife with a cold or septic focus should be on duty.

PROMOTION OF BREAST FEEDING

In order to succeed, the mother must want to breast feed. Normally the baby is allowed to suck within 6 hours of birth. The midwife may have to help ensure that the mother is in a comfortable position and that the baby also is comfortable and able to breathe freely whilst sucking. The baby must grasp the whole areolar area

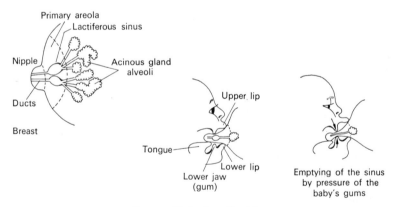

FIG. 12.4 Mechanism of sucking

and not just the nipple. In the early puerperium the breasts secrete colostrum and mature milk takes a few weeks to appear. At first the quantity is small. Therefore at first the baby should only suck for a few minutes and very gradually the feeding time is increased to a maximum of 10 minutes on each breast. At first the baby normally wants to suck frequently and demand feeding is best, but the interval between feeds should not exceed 4 hours, except possibly at night.

If engorgement of the breasts occurs the doctor may order one dose of stilboestrol (3–5 mg orally). If lactation is to succeed and infection be avoided, the nipples must not be allowed to crack.

Some mothers produce surplus milk and they should be taught how to hand express the surplus after their baby has fed. (In hospital an electric humilactor can be used.) This surplus milk is collected by regional breast milk banks and is most useful for sick or low weight babies. Careful washing of the nipples is important to prevent infection.

Occasionally breast feeding is unwise because of a serious medical condition or because the mother's nipples are badly inverted (this is rare). If the baby is still-born lactation must be suppressed. Many mothers, though capable, just refuse to breast feed. These mothers are usually of low intelligence and live under poor social conditions. The production of milk can be suppressed by the use of oestrogens; the usual being stilboestrol 5 mg tds for 5 days. Recently a risk of thrombosis has been attributed to stilboestrol and there is now some doubt if oestrogens are really necessary. Stilboestrol has been prescribed by doctors without real thought. They have been prescribed when a mother has insufficient milk for her baby. At this time oestrogens are unnecessary. If the baby does not suck, milk will not be produced. For a few days any surplus milk can be expressed by the mother. Midwives and Health Visitors must discourage mothers from rushing to their doctor for stilboestrol.

Estrovis is probably better than stilboestrol in preventing milk formation, but must be given within 6 hours of delivery to be effective. Probably hormones are not really necessary. With a firm supportive brassière most women will experience little discomfort. To the few who do, a diuretic such as lasix can be prescribed by the doctor.

Successful lactation does frequently require patience, help and encouragement by the midwife. Unfortunately many young midwives (and doctors) lack training in this aspect of midwifery. Too many breast fed babies are offered complementary cow's milk bottle feeds during the early days of life. Are these necessary?

When the baby is artificially fed the midwife must instruct the mother in the preparation of a suitable milk feed (see 'care of baby' (page 76)).

EDUCATION OF THE MOTHER IN THE MANAGEMENT OF HER BABY

The mother should be encouraged early to know when her baby is hungry. The mother should change her baby's napkins and know what normal stools should look like. She should be taught how to bath her baby and treat the skin folds.

Examinations

Initial examination. It is customary for a doctor to examine a mother about 8 to 10 days after delivery, before she is discharged from hospital, and before a midwife leaves in a home delivery. This examination includes a general check on the patient's blood pressure, urine and haemoglobin. A vaginal examination is valuable to assess accurately the size of the uterus and to ensure that the cervix has closed down, and that there is no abnormality in the fornices. The perineum should have healed if sutured and all unabsorbable sutures been removed. The tone of the pelvic floor muscles should be checked. The patient should be encouraged to continue pelvic floor exercises for some months. The patient's legs are inspected for varicose veins and any evidence of thrombosis. The breasts are checked. The patient must be encouraged to have a further postnatal examination when the baby is about 6 weeks old.

Futher postnatal examination. A history of both mother and baby is taken including an enquiry about lactation.

The patient's weight is recorded and a sample of urine tested for protein, glucose and pus. The blood pressure is taken and haemoglobin checked (if in the early puerperium the haemoglobin was below 80 per cent—11·5 g).

Examination includes inspection of the mother's breasts and abdominal muscular tone. The vulva is inspected for any abnormal discharge or prolapse, and to ensure that the perineum is satisfactory. The doctor will make a vaginal examination to check that the uterus is normal in size and position and also the appendages. A speculum is inserted for the inspection of the cervix to ensure that the external os looks normal. It is usual to take cervical smear tests at this time to exclude cancer. The patient's anus is inspected to exclude haemorrhoids and an anal fissure. The patient's legs are inspected for oedema and varicose veins.

Treatment may be necessary for the cervix—an erosion should be cauterised. If the uterus is retroverted, the patient should be advised regarding posture in bed and instructed to have the uterine position checked early in a subsequent pregnancy. If the pelvic floor muscles are not normal, continuing exercises are essential.

The patient should be advised regarding future deliveries, whether or not a hospital confinement is necessary. If the mother requires birth control advice she should be told how to obtain this.

Further visits may be necessary if the blood pressure is raised or the urine is abnormal. If the cervix is eroded the patient should be examined again, usually in about 6 week's time.

The object of the postnatal examination is to leave mothers in good health and ready for further conception, if desired.

13 DISEASES AFFECTING PREGNANCY

CARDIAC DISEASE

At the age of pregnancy the usual cardiac lesion will be a congenital abnormality or mitral stenosis following rheumatic fever, recurrent tonsillitis, or influenza. Usually the patient will know that she has a cardiac lesion, but sometimes the doctor will discover one on the first routine medical examination.

Because the heart requires to work harder than usual during pregnancy, there is a risk of cardiac failure. The patient should be advised to secure adequate rest, this may mean stopping any heavy work. She must be under the care of a consultant obstetrician and it is wise to refer her to a heart specialist. The maximum strain on the heart is between the 28th and 36th weeks of pregnancy. If the patient is unable to achieve adequate rest at home, she should be offered a hospital bed. The heart condition will deteriorate if she is allowed to become anaemic or if she should develop bronchitis or toxaemia or any infection. Should heart failure occur, treatment with digitalis is indicated. Very rarely an emergency heart operation is deemed to be necessary, for instance if the patient has haemoptysis or severe orthopnoea.

A vaginal delivery is preferable to a Caesarean Section, but all cardiac patients should be delivered in hospital. A difficult delivery should be avoided. It is wise for labour to start in hospital and therefore it is customary to admit patients with cardiac disease about one week before term; fortunately the baby is usually fairly small.

The first stage of labour should not strain the heart. The usual sedation is adequate. In the second stage the patient must be discouraged from pushing. A doctor should be present. Unless the fetus advances well, the doctor should deliver the baby with forceps under pudendal local anaesthesia. The third stage is the most serious for such cases because with the delivery of the placenta there is a sudden change in blood volume. If possible the third stage should be as normal as possible, oxytoxic drugs being avoided unless haemorrhage occurs. The patient must be watched carefully for at least 2 hours from the time of delivery and not moved. The doctor may give antibiotics prophylactically because bacterial endocarditis can occur around the time of delivery.

In the puerperium the patient should not be too active. If she wants to breast feed she can (unless there has been cardiac failure). Breast feeding is easier than preparing artificial feeds at home, unless she has adequate help. She should remain in hospital for at least 10 days, and a home help will be valuable after she has been discharged from hospital.

A patient with a heart lesion should limit her family to two or three children and she should be advised about birth control when she attends the postnatal clinic. Sterilisation may be considered.

TUBERCULOSIS

Any woman with known *pulmonary tuberculosis* should be advised to refrain from becoming pregnant until her lung condition has healed: this means 2 years after the disease has become quiescent.

Fortunately pulmonary tuberculosis has become less common. The only certain method of diagnosis is by chest X-ray. This investigation is recommended during each pregnancy in immigrants and annually if the woman is BCG negative or living in poor social conditions. Otherwise, it is only necessary if the patient has not had a chest X-ray within 3 years. Mass X-ray centres use suitable equipment so that the foetus is not at risk. Midwives must ensure that their patients have this X-ray.

If pulmonary tuberculosis is diagnosed, the patient should receive the appropriate drugs, otherwise she will tend to abort or go into premature labour. Unless she can obtain adequate rest at home she will be admitted to a chest hospital. Tubercle bacilli are relatively large and therefore fail to pass from the maternal to fetal bloodstream, unless the placenta is affected by a tuberculoma. This is very rare. Antituberculous drugs pass to the fetus and can cause trouble. Streptomycin may affect the hearing of the baby but usually this is not severe. Isoniazid may increase the risk of maternal megaloblastic anaemia. The delivery should be in hospital. The first stage is conducted as usual. The patient should refrain from pushing during the second stage and a doctor should be present. It is important to minimise blood loss, therefore the doctor will usually give ergometrine 0·5 mg IV after the baby is born.

If the mother has a positive sputum or her lesion is recently active, lactation should be suppressed if necessary with lasix 120 mgm. She may have to return to the chest hospital to complete her treatment. Calcium is required for the healing of her lung lesion and also for lactation.

It is wise for the baby to be vaccinated with BCG prior to coming under the mother's care. Whilst immunity is developing, the baby may have to be separated from its mother. This is essential if the mother's sputum is still positive.

Genital Tuberculosis. The Fallopian tubes may become infected by a bloodstream spread of tubercle bacilli from a primary lung lesion. Unless recognised and treated early, the Fallopian tubes become blocked and the woman becomes sterile. Early treatment can prevent this blockage. Infection can arise after a miscarriage or labour. Sometimes, even with treatment, the infected tube prevents a fertilised ovum from reaching the uterus and an ectopic pregnancy ensues. When the Fallopian tube is infected, the tubercle bacilli pass into the endometrium and can be recognised in uterine curettings, sometimes on histological examination; but more often after innoculating a guinea pig and examining the animal later for tuberculosis.

Routine chest X-ray of adolescent girls should reveal any pulmonary tuberculous lesion and with treatment prevent genital infection. Routine skin testing for tuberculosis will indicate those girls who have no resistance to tuberculosis. Vaccination with BCG should be given to create resistance.

If menstrual periods are irregular or bleeding excessive following a delivery or miscarriage, uterine curettings should be examined for tuberculosis.

Renal tuberculosis. One or both kidneys can be affected, usually by a bloodstream spread from a primary lung lesion. The urine will contain pus cells, sometimes red blood corpuscles and protein. If the urine is cultured none of the usual organisms, e.g. *E. coli* are cultured. The pus cells persist after the usual antibiotic therapy.

If a woman with a tuberculous kidney becomes pregnant, the results for her and her baby can be serious. Consequently, any pregnant woman with pus in her urine must be fully investigated. If, on culture of the urine, no organisms are grown, the urine should be injected into a guinea pig. The patient's renal function must be tested. Active anti-tuberculous treatment must be given if indicated. With poor functioning kidneys, diagnosed in early pregnancy, the patient may require a therapeutic abortion.

Osseous tuberculosis. Bones are usually affected by the bovine type of tuberculosis. Since milk is now pasteurised and tuberculin free cattle reared, the disease is, fortunately, rare. If spinal disease occurs before puberty, the pelvis may be asymmetrical. Active spinal disease is rarely seen in a pregnant woman, because she will, as a rule, be receiving tuberculosis treatment in a plaster jacket. Calcium is essential for healing of the tuberculous and a pregnancy would be detrimental.

CHOREA (St. Vitus's dance)

This disease is characterised by incoordinate, non-purposive movements. Chorea is a possible complication of rheumatic disease, but fortunately is not common. About one-third of choreic patients also have a heart lesion. Pregnancy tends to aggravate the condition and miscarriages are common. Patients with chorea must be delivered in hospital under consultant care. Puerperal psychosis is fairly frequent. Patients with chorea should be advised to limit the number of children they have.

THYROID DISEASE

(1) *Myxoedema* (hypothyroidism). Patients with myxoedema tend to be overweight with poor hair growth and a dry skin. Their menstrual periods are often irregular and infertility is common. If conception occurs, miscarriages are common unless the patient's condition is recognised early and adequate thyroid therapy is given.

(2) *Goitre* (hyperthyroidism). The thyroid gland is enlarged and overactive. The patient frequently has a rapid pulse rate, fine tremor of the fingers, sometimes exophthalmos and is thin with a warm skin. Hypertension is common. Medical treatment is effective, but during pregnancy the drugs pass through the placenta to the developing fetus and can cause goitre in the new-born baby. In the early puerperium the mother may develop a thyroid crisis. Operative surgery may be advisable in cases of severe thyrotoxicosis during pregnancy.

During pregnancy the investigation of thyroid function is difficult. In pregnancy there is a normal rise in the metabolic rate and the level of blood cholesterols also rises. Radioactive iodine investigation can be harmful to the fetus.

VENEREAL DISEASES

Veneral diseases are those passed from man to woman or vice versa at intercourse.

(1) *Syphilis.* The syphilitic spirochaete is relatively large, but attacks placental tissue and therefore passes from maternal to fetal blood. The initial lesion in the female is a painless indurated ulcer at the vulva. From this a smear will reveal the spirochaete on special examination with a ground-glass microscope. The next

phase is invasion of the bloodstream giving a transient rash and a positive Wassermann blood reaction. Later effects are gumma in various organs and the (tertiary phase) involvement of the cerebrospinal fluid.

Unless syphilis is treated early in pregnancy, the fetus will abort or be still-born. Milder infections can give a live birth, but the baby tends to be snuffling and fails to thrive normally. The baby's skin has a copper-coloured rash on the soles of the feet and the palms of the hand. The baby can develop a syphilitic eye lesion (keratitis) and joint epiphysitis, also bowing of the legs.

Because syphilis is serious, it is necessary to test every pregnant woman's blood by a Wassermann or comparable test, as early as possible in pregnancy. Syphilis can be readily treated with penicillin.

(2) *Gonorrhoea*. Gonococci are difficult to culture. The organism invades glands and in a female may cause a salpingitis and joint pain. There is usually a profuse vaginal discharge and sometimes a pyrexia develops. Unless gonorrhoea is recognised and treated during pregnancy, the baby's eyes may become infected during delivery, and this can lead to blindness without correct treatment.

Midwives must examine patients during pregnancy for a vaginal discharge, not just relying on the history. If a discharge is seen, the patient must be referred to a doctor who will take a vaginal swab for culture. Gonorrhoea responds as a rule, quite readily to penicillin therapy.

Patients with syphilis and gonorrhoea are usually referred to a special veneral disease clinic so that contacts can also be investigated and, if need be, treated.

(3) *Trichomonas vaginitis*. This is caused by a flagellate organism, easily recognised on microscopic examination. This organism causes a typical yellow, frothy, irritating vaginal discharge in the female. In the male there are no symptoms. Trichomonas infection is common during pregnancy because of the altered acidity of the vagina.

If a midwife notices any abnormal vaginal discharge she must refer the patient to a doctor. The treatment for trichomonas is usually by Flagyl tablets: these should be taken by the man as well as the woman. Trichomonas does not seem to affect the fetus and the new-born baby, except that an infected vagina may attract secondary infection with pathogenic organisms.

Another common vaginal discharge in pregnancy is due to thrush (monilia). This responds to nystatin pessaries. If the mother is untreated the baby may develop thrush after delivery, especially of the mouth, but thrush can pass lower in the intestinal tract. Skin thrush can occur.

Any of the other pathogenic organisms can invade the vagina during pregnancy. Therefore every abnormal vaginal discharge should be investigated and treated. Numerous types of pessary are available.

PYELONEPHRITIS

Pyelitis is inflammation of the pelvis of the kidney. In reality the infection usually involves renal tissue as well and therefore the condition is really a pyelonephritis. The usual causal organism is the bacillus *E. coli*, but other organisms can be involved.

Pyelonephritis is common during pregnancy. especially on the right side, because of stasis of urine due to compression of the ureter against the pelvic brim by the growing uterus. Unless the infection is recognised early and treated, the infection can become chronic with serious results. The disease tends to be symptomless, initially because the ureters being dilated during pregnancy prevent typical renal colic. In acute cases pyrexia may develop. Pyelonephritis may precipitate a premature labour.

At every antenatal examination, the midwife must suspect infection if the urine appears cloudy or has an offensive odour. In such cases medical aid must be sought If pyclitis is suspected the patient should be referred to hospital. A midstream specimen of urine is sent for microscopic examination and culture. Patients with pyelitis benefit from hospital treatment. Usually a short course of sulphonamides (e.g. gantrisin) will be given and the patient encouraged to take plenty of fluids. Prolonged therapy should be avoided because the fetus will also receive the drug.

If the urine fails to clear a renal calculus must be suspected: persistent pus may be due to tuberculosis. Full renal function tests may be necessary.

ANAEMIA IN PREGNANCY

This is common and several different types are recognised:

(1) *Iron deficiency*. This is the most common variety and is shown by a fall in the haemoglobin (Hb). Because of the increased blood volume, an Hb count of 80 per cent (11·5 g) is accepted as normal, although some authorities consider 75 per cent (10·5 g) to be more realistic. Iron is saved because of the cessation of menstrual bleeding, but the fetus requires iron and stores iron in its liver, especially during the last four weeks. Many obstetricians prescribe routine iron throughout pregnancy, but iron can upset the patient's digestion and it is still necessary to check her haemoglobin. A good iron-containing diet seems more rational. Iron can be lost from bleeding. During pregnancy bleeding may occur from the vagina, rectum or nose. The latter may be due to a lowering of prothrombin. Midwives should ensure that their patients have regular haemoglobin estimations. If the result is below 80 per cent (11·59) medical aid must be sought.

(2) *Megaloblastic anaemia* is due to a low folic acid level. Extra folic acid is required in pregnancy because of increased metabolism. The typical megaloblastic cells are difficult to find in the circulating blood. An examination of the bone marrow will prove the condition. Megaloblastic anaemia is a likely diagnosis when an anaemic patient fails to respond to iron therapy.

Some obstetrians prescribe routine folic acid with iron during pregnancy. It is interesting that the need for folic acid becomes greater if routine iron is given.

Megaloblastic anaemia can cause a sore tongue, subcuticular haemorrhages and diarrhoea. Megaloblastic anaemia may be precipitated by drugs such as isoniazid, phenobarbitone and others used in the treatment of epilepsy.

(3) *Aplastic anaemia*. If this is a congenital anomaly the outlook is serious. Metals can be responsible, e.g. gold, lead and many others. Withdrawal of the offending substance can be curative. Most patients will require blood transfusions.

(4) *Haemoglobinopathies*. Numerous haemoglobin abnormalities have been described. The more common include:

Sickle cell anaemia. This occurs almost exclusively in the negro race. Abnormal sickle cells can be seen in the circulating blood when special stains are used. Besides anaemia, a pyrexia can occur, also joint pain and jaundice. Reduced oxygen can precipitate a fatal crisis, therefore it is important that the anomaly is known to the anaesthetist who may be required to give the patient a general anaesthetic. If the anaemia is severe, blood transfusions may be required.

Thalassaemia (Cooley's anaemia). This is a hereditary defect of mediterranean races in which the fetal type of haemoglobin persists. Typical 'target cells' can be found in the blood. If both parents have this trait they are unlikely to produce children who live to adulthood.

(5) *Anaemia* is common in the presence of infection, particularly pyelitis. The infection must be treated before the anaemia will improve.

(6) *Leukaemia* is rare in the child-bearing age group, but will be revealed on examining a blood film. Leukaemia is very serious.

Anaemia can cause miscarriages, premature labours, antepartum haemorrhage and even fetal death. The patient (especially with an iron deficiency) may have few symptoms until the Hb falls to a low level. She may feel tired and have headaches. During labour an anaemic patient, even with a reasonably normal blood loss, may become shocked and a postpartum haemorrhage can be fatal.

It is imperative to recognise anaemia during pregnancy, whilst there is time for full investigation and treatment. This may require admission to an antenatal ward.

Management. If a pregnant woman's Hb falls below 80 per cent (11·5 g), the doctor, after ascertaining that there is no obvious bleeding, and advising the patient regarding diet, will usually prescribe oral iron. The cheapest effective tablets are ferrous sulphate 200 mg t.d.s. taken with meals. The Hb will be checked at the patient's next routine antenatal examination. If the Hb has failed to rise and the patient has been taking iron tablets, folic acid 5 mg daily is usually prescribed. If the Hb falls below 70 per cent the patient should be admitted for the following examinations:

(1) Serum iron level.

(2) Stools (3 specimens) sent for examination for occult blood and parasites.

(3) Urine. Mid-stream specimen for a bacterial count and culture.

(4) A blood film examination to exclude sickle and target cells (in the appropriate races) and leukaemia.

(5) Very rarely, if all the above tests prove to be normal, special investigations for an enzyme deficiency such as glucose phosphate hydrogenase or B_{12} is done.

The treatment depends on the results of these investigations. If the serum iron is low, it can be failure of normal iron absorption and the doctor can give parenteral iron. This is usually by a continuous imferon intravenous drip, otherwise by intramuscular injections of jectofer.

GLYCOSURIA DURING PREGNANCY

This is relatively common and may be of two types:

(1) *Renal glycosuria.* In this type, the urine contains glucose, although the blood sugar remains normal The cause is thought to be an alteration in hormones. Renal glycosuria has no pathological significance, except the patient should take adequate sugar to prevent symptoms of hypoglycaemia.

(2) *Diabetic or prediabetic glycosuria.* Diabetes may become manifest for the first time during the stress of a pregnancy. Patients who will become diabetic in later life may show the first signs during a pregnancy. In diabetes a blood sugar curve reaches abnormally high levels.

In prediabetes the blood sugar curve shows slow glucose absorption and the blood sugar after 2 hours remains over 100 mg (6 m|mol S.I. units) per litre. In both diabetes and prediabetes the fetus tends to grow abnormally large. It may die in utero near term or cause a difficult delivery.

The midwife's duty is to test the pregnant woman's urine for glucose at each examination. The clinistix test is usually used, but this gives many false positive results. If a clinistix test is positive, the tablet clinitest should be used. If this is positive, the midwife must seek medical aid and the doctor should refer the patient to hospital where a glucose tolerance test can be done.

If the glucose tolerance test is normal or, as is often the case, low, the patient should be encouraged to have a normal carbohydrate diet. She can be reassured that everything is normal.

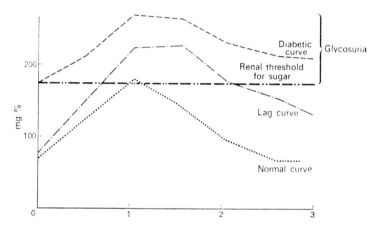

FIG. 13.1 Glucose tolerance test

If the glucose tolerance test reveals a true diabetic curve, the patient should be referred to a consultant physician. Insulin or oral preparations may be prescribed together with a restricted carbohydrate diet. Diabetic patients may complain of excessive thirst or skin irritation.

Where the blood sugar test reveals a 'lag curve' no drugs are necessary, but if overweight the patient will benefit by reducing her carbohydrate intake.

Diabetic and prediabetic patients should have labour induced about the 38th week. A vaginal delivery (provided labour is not prolonged) is preferable to a Caesarean Section. Delivery must be in hospital. The baby may require special care as there is an increased risk of respiratory complications.

Diabetes tends to be a familial disease, therefore the family history should be carefully investigated. An untreated diabetic may be relatively infertile or tend to miscarry in early pregnancy. A diabetic should limit her family as every pregnancy tends to worsen the condition. Sterilisation may be advisable.

OTHER DISEASES

There are some diseases, fortunately rare, which may affect a pregnant women without causing symptoms to her, but which are dangerous to the fetus. Such diseases include:

(1) *Toxoplasmosis*. The protozoon *Toxoplasma gondii* is common in rodents, especially rabbits, and birds. If a pregnant woman becomes infected, fetal death may occur and premature labour is common. The baby may show signs of hydrocephaly, icterus, an enlarged spleen and liver, rashes, pyrexia or chorioretinitis—serological dye tests prove the diagnosis. Subsequent children will not be affected.

(2) *Cytomegalic inclusion disease*. This virus does not affect the adult woman but during pregnancy will cross the placenta affecting the fetus. Still-births and premature deliveries are common. The baby may have convulsions, a large liver and spleen, thrombopaenic purpura, icterus and anaemia. Characteristic intranuclear and intracytoplasmic inclusion bodies are present in the fetal kidneys and liver. The virus can be cultured from the urine and saliva. If the baby survives, microcephaly is common and the child may be mentally retarded.

DRUG ADDICTION

Heroin has a low molecular weight and passes through the placenta to the fetus. Fetal complications have been described in American literature. Pregnant women on heroin have an increased incidence of abortions, still-births and premature labours. Such women tend to obtain little antenatal care and advice. Toxaemia is common and also venereal disease. Their diet is usually inadequate.

The baby may show evidence of heroin withdrawal during the early days of life. This includes asphyxia, cerebral irritation and gastrointestinal disturbances. Congenital abnormalities are fairly common, and phenylketonuria is occasionally present. There is little published evidence concerning the 'softer' drugs (cannabis, amphetamine etc.).

MISCARRIAGES OR ABORTIONS (the terms are synonymous)

A miscarriage means the delivery of a fetus and membranes before the 28th week of pregnancy, the fetus failing to breathe. The patient undergoes a miniature labour with cervical dilatation and pain. The most common time for a miscarriage to occur is about the 12th week.

Frequently, no cause can be determined, although there are many possible factors:
(a) *Paternal*. Poor quality of the spermatozoon may cause a miscarriage. Therefore where recurrent miscarriages occur, the husband should have his seminal fluid examined. If the husband has syphilis, he will infect his wife and this may lead to a miscarriage.
(b) *Fetal*. Recent work has shown that many early aborted fetuses are abnormal. Consequently it is important to have the fetus examined by a pathologist. Abnormalities of the placenta (e.g. hydatidiform mole) or a tumour (e.g. haemangioma) tend to interrupt pregnancy.
(c) *Maternal*. Several general diseases tend to cause miscarriages, such as hypertension, chronic nephritis or pyelonephritis, diabetes, thyroid abnormalities, severe heart disease or any pyrexial illness. An abdominal operation or old abdominal adhesions may also be responsible for a miscarriage.

Any uterine abnormality such as a bicornuate uterus, fibroids or retroversion are possible causes. A lax cervix with incompetent circular muscles around the internal os will cause a miscarriage, usually rather late in pregnancy. The ovaries may produce inadequate hormones for a pregnancy to continue, but the value of hormone therapy in preventing miscarriages is still under debate.

Adequate vitamins are essential in pregnancy and lack of these (as has been shown in animal experiments) may well be responsible for some miscarriages. Recent work suggests that a deficiency of folic acid may be a cause of miscarriage.

Abnormal embedding of the ovum, e.g. in the lower uterine segment (placenta praevia), may account for some miscarriages. A few miscarriages may be caused by violent exercise, e.g. horse riding or using a treadle machine. Car accidents are a modern cause. Certain drugs can be responsible for miscarriage such as lead, quinine and ergot.

Miscarriages may occur spontaneously or be induced, the latter either illegally for personal reasons (by the patient or some other person) or for therapeutic reasons by a doctor.

Types of Miscarriage

Miscarriages may be threatened or inevitable. A *threatened* miscarriage is shown by bleeding and sometimes a little pain, but the cervix remains closed. A pregnant woman should call a midwife or doctor if any bleeding occurs. The patient should be sent to hospital or kept in bed at home. Everything she passes vaginally must be saved. Strict bed rest is the best treatment. A sedative may be useful. If bleeding has been at all severe hospital treatment is advised. Blood should be sent for cross-matching in case a transfusion is required. The patient's haemoglobin should be checked. Any possible cause of the threatened miscarriage must be investigated. The patient should remain in bed until there has been no bleeding for one week. Thereafter she should avoid intercourse for at least six weeks and should rest.

After threatened miscarriages many pregnancies will continue successfully to term, but a hospital delivery is advisable. There is a slightly increased fetal risk.

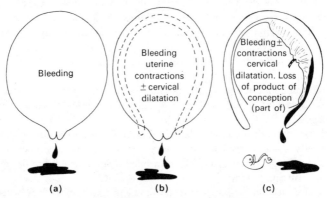

FIG. 14.1 Types of abortion: (a) threatened, (b) inevitable, (c) incomplete

The fetus has about a 4 per cent greater chance of being abnormal than in a pregnancy without bleeding.

When the cervix dilates a miscarriage is *inevitable*. The products may be completely expelled, but frequently placental tissue is retained (*incomplete miscarriage*) giving risk of haemorrhage (sometimes severe) and of sepsis. When miscarriage is inevitable, an enema can be given to hasten the miscarriage.

If the miscarriage is incomplete, the patient may require an anaesthetic and curettage of the uterus after dilating the cervix. Because a pregnant uterus is soft, only a blunt curette must be used to avoid perforation of the uterus and dilatation must be gentle to prevent tearing of the cervix. It is important to check that the fetus and all membrane and placental tissue are passed. All tissue should be examined by a pathologist.

The main risks after a miscarriage are haemorrhage and sepsis.

Other types of miscarriage include:

(1) *Missed Abortion*. For some reason the fetus dies and remains in utero. When this occurs, symptoms of pregnancy retrogress. If fetal movements have been felt by the patient, they now cease. The fundal height shrinks. The breasts may secrete milk. After about two weeks the urine ceases to contain gonadotrophic hormones and a pregnancy urine test becomes negative. Occasionally hypofibrinogenaemia occurs.

To encourage the uterus to expel a dead fetus, the doctor may give fairly high doses of pitocin (or syntocinon). An alternative, probably better method, is to use prostaglandin (prostin E_2) intravenously. Occasionally there is a slight inflammatory reaction on the arm but this is never serious.

(2) *Ectopic Pregnancy.* This means the fertilised ovum fails to reach the uterus. A tubal pregnancy usually results. Early symptoms are pain in an iliac fossa. Occasionally, the enlarged tube can be felt by the doctor on vaginal examination, and touching the cervix causes some pain. The patient usually gives a history of irregular bleeding or a dark brown discharge.

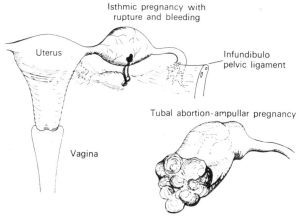

FIG. 14.2 Ectopic pregnancy

The cause of an ectopic pregnancy is usually previous disease of the Fallopian tube as may occur during the puerperium from sepsis, or salpingitis due to gonorrhoea or tuberculosis.

The Fallopian tube is unable to expand much. Therefore unless the fertilised ovum passes back into the peritoneal cavity, the tube will rupture. If the tear occurs in the lower part of the tube, the ovum may pass into the Pouch of Douglas. With rupture the patient generally experiences some pain and later backache. If the tear is through the upper surface of the tube, bleeding can be severe and the patient presents as an acute abdominal crisis. She will become shocked and pale. Early laparotomy and blood transfusion are necessary to control haemorrhage. Usually the tube has to be sacrificed.

Very occasionally the ovum, after leaving the tube, receives nourishment in the peritoneal cavity from the omentum and continues to grow. Full term can be reached. Then signs of labour occur but the cervix will not dilate. Fetal parts are felt abnormally easily through the abdominal wall. A laparotomy is necessary for delivery. It may be very difficult to detach the placenta from the omentum. Occasionally, the placenta has to be left in situ to be absorbed.

If a tubal pregnancy is diagnosed early, a laparotomy should be done and the fetus with placental tissues removed. The diagnosis can be difficult. Laparoscopic examination by a skilled doctor can be very helpful.

(3) *Hydatidiform mole.* Occasionally the chorionic villi become cystic, secrete excess gonadotrophic hormones and prevent fetal growth. The excess villi cause abnormal growth of the uterus during the early weeks of pregnancy and the

uterus feels abnormally soft. The chorionic villi can penetrate into the uterine wall, even reaching the peritoneal surface. Typically, some blood and cystic villi are expelled vaginally. This discharge is described as 'white currants in red currant juice'. This can be a serious condition leading to a highly malignant chorionepithelioma of the uterus.

Bleeding in early pregnancy and an abnormally large soft uterus must make one suspect a hydatidiform mole. A quantitative pregnancy urine test may confirm the diagnosis. Treatment depends upon the age and parity of the patient. If she is nearing 40 and has had her desired family, hysterectomy is best. In a younger woman, the uterus should be evacuated by a D and C (dilatation of the cervix

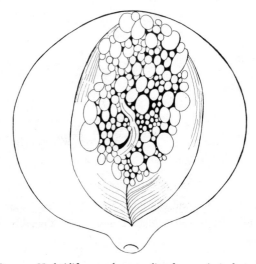

FIG. 14.3 Hydatidiform mole protruding from an incised uterus

and uterine curettage). This may be accompanied by heavy bleeding and it may be difficult to remove all chorionic tissue. Gonadotrophic urinary tests must be repeated monthly for 6 months and then about every 2 months up to 2 years to ensure that active tissue has not been left to form a chorionepithelioma.

The Abortion Act passed in April 1968 was designed to reduce the number of illegal abortions. A suitably qualified doctor can now perform an abortion for the following reasons, but only after a second doctor (usually the patient's general practitioner) agrees:

(a) When the continuance of the pregnancy would involve risk to the life of the pregnant woman greater than if the pregnancy were terminated.

(b) When the continuance of the pregnancy would involve risk of injury to the physical or mental health of the pregnant woman, greater than if the pregnancy were terminated.

(c) When the continuance of the pregnancy would involve risk of injury to the physical or mental health of the existing child(ren) of the family of the pregnant woman, greater than if the pregnancy were terminated.

(d) When there is a substantial risk that if the child were born it would suffer from such physical or mental abnormalities as to be seriously handicapped.

After an abortion the patient should receive contraceptive advice.

HYPEREMESIS GRAVIDARUM

Vomiting before breakfast is fairly common during the first three months of pregnancy. Occasionally vomiting persists throughout the day and the condition is termed hyperemesis. Vomiting in pregnancy soon causes ketosis and later loss in weight, alteration in blood electrolytes, proteinuria and jaundice. The disease can but should not be fatal.

If a pregnant woman complains of vomiting, her urine must be tested for acetone. If this is found, the midwife must seek medical aid and the doctor should refer the patient to hospital for admission. Early treatment gives excellent results. If ketosis has been present for some time prior to treatment, relapses are frequent. In the old days, a therapeutic abortion was sometimes necessary.

Medical treatment consists of giving intravenous glucose. About 200 ml of 20 per cent dextrose should combat ketosis, but if the patient is dehydrated a continuous drip of 5 per cent glucose saline may be required, and the blood electrolytes must be checked. The doctor will exclude other causes for vomiting, e.g. pyelitis, any intestinal lesion or even a cerebral lesion. If the patient is worried, the doctor will usually prescribe a sedative, e.g. sol. luminal 180 mg IM (phenobarbitone).

Nursing care is very important. The patient requires reassurance. If she can retain fluids by mouth, small frequent glucose drinks should be given. When she feels hungry, small dry meals should be given with drinks between meals. Her urinary output should be measured, and the urine tested daily for acetone, protein and bile. Vitamin B_1 helps protein and carbohydrate metabolism and may be prescribed by the doctor. When vomiting has ceased, the patient should gradually return to a normal diet. It is wise to keep her in hospital for about one week after vomiting has ceased. Too early a discharge home (where she will as a rule have to cook) may lead to a relapse.

Hyperemesis is probably caused by a low blood sugar due to the alteration of hormones with pregnancy. It is especially common in a multiple pregnancy and with a hydatidiform mole. Some women vomit more readily than others, even when not pregnant. After the third month of pregnancy hyperemesis is rare. Numerous drugs have been recommended, most of doubtful value and some such as thalidomide have proved to affect normal fetal development. All drugs, especially at this vital stage of fetal development should be avoided.

RETROVERTED UTERUS

Some women are born with a retroverted uterus and in some the uterus becomes retroverted after childbirth. Retroversion makes conception more difficult. For a pregnancy to continue the uterine fundus must become anteverted by the 12th week in order to rise into the abdomen. A retroverted uterus may spontaneously rectify its position but miscarriages are frequent. Another possibility is that the pregnant uterus remains incarcerated in the pelvis. Very rarely sacculation of a portion of the anterior wall occurs and the sac rises into the abdomen with the fetus. A full term pregnancy, in such a case, is unlikely to occur, and there is a real danger that the thin uterine sac will rupture. Consequently, early diagnosis and correction of a retroverted gravid uterus is important.

The earliest symptom is backache. Later (about the 12th week) there may be difficulty with micturition leading to a dribbling overflow from a full bladder. If incarceration occurs pain is severe. Many cases of retroversion are found accidentally when the doctor performs a vaginal examination to confirm a suspected early

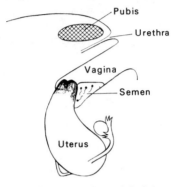

FIG. 14.4 Retroversion: conception is difficult because cervix is pointing away from pool of semen

pregnancy. When a retroverted uterus has been found, the position should be corrected. Frequently this is easily done bimanually and many doctors will insert a Hodge pessary to ensure that the uterus will remain anteverted. The pessary should be removed after the 14th week of pregnancy. If replacement is at all difficult the

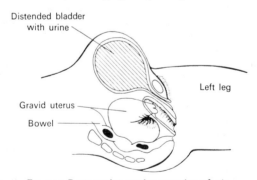

FIG. 14.5 Retroversion causing retention of urine

patient should be admitted to hospital for postural therapy. This means raising the foot of the bed about 1½ feet, and encouraging the patient to lie prone or on her side. If incarceration has occurred, the bladder may have to be emptied by catheterization. The urine will, as a rule, be infected and in these cases an appropriate antibiotic will be prescribed by the doctor.

If the uterus fails to become anteverted after postural treatment, it may have to be manipulated forward under a general anaesthetic. This is rarely necessary.

TOXAEMIA

This is probably the most important antenatal complication, accounting for a high proportion of fetal and also maternal deaths. The term may be a misnomer but a better one is still awaited.

Usually four types are described:

(1) Pre-eclampsia
(2) Hypertensive toxaemia
(3) Nephritic toxaemia
(4) Acute yellow atrophy of the liver

(1) Pre-eclampsia

The three cardinal signs are oedema, a raised blood pressure and proteinuria. Despite a great deal of research, the exact cause is still uncertain, but with early diagnosis serious complications can usually be avoided. Characteristically, a patient begins her pregnancy with a normal blood pressure, i.e. 130/80 mm Hg or less and with no protein in the urine.

Pre-eclampsia is most common in a first pregnancy, but is also common in a twin or multiple pregnancy. Signs rarely occur before the 28th week unless a hydatidiform mole is present. Hydramnios and diabetes can precipitate toxaemia.

The earliest sign is usually oedema, preceded often by an excessive gain in weight (more than 1 lb (482 g) per week). Usually the blood pressure rises and later protein appears in the urine. Although the cause is still debatable, the placenta is usually infarcted. There is increased secretion of urinary gonadotrophins and a reduction of oestrogens and progesterone. The blood pressure probably rises because of a vascular spasm. This spasm causes renal ischaemia, which can account for the proteinuria. The oedema is due to an upset in sodium water balance. In fatal cases, the liver shows subcapsular haemorrhages and is abnormally yellow. This may cause jaundice and bile in the urine. The brain is oedematous and ischaemic. The kidneys show oedema of the basement membrane. Placental infarcts interfere with fetal nutrition and as a consequence the fetal weight is below average. In severe cases, the fetus may be deprived of adequate oxygen and die in utero. The abnormal infarcted placenta may separate early causing an antepartum or intrapartum (during labour) bleeding. In severe cases the patient may develop eclamptic fits.

Management. Although pre-eclampsia cannot, with our present knowledge, be prevented, early diagnosis and careful management should prevent many of the serious complications. Midwives can often diagnose the condition early. At every antenatal examination, the patient's weight and blood pressure must be recorded. The urine must be tested for protein. The presence of oedema should be noted. If the midwife finds an excessive weight gain or oedema, without signs of toxaemia, the midwife should advise the patient to obtain extra rest and to restrict her salt intake. The patient should be examined again within one week. When the blood pressure rises (diastolic of 90 mm Hg or more) the doctor should be informed. The doctor should refer a patient to hospital and the patient be admitted when:

(a) There is oedema and the diastolic BP has reached 90 mm Hg or above.
(b) The diastolic blood pressure reaches 100 mm Hg, without oedema.
(c) Every case when protein occurs in the urine.

It behoves Maternity Hospitals to provide adequate antenatal beds to cater for these admissions. The reason for hospital admission is to provide constant observation in order to detect fetal or maternal danger. Suitable charts are used to record the daily fluid intake and urinary output. The urine is tested for protein daily, in addition an Esbach estimation of the quantity of protein passed during 24 hours is made. The blood pressure should be recorded twice daily, but when the diastolic reading exceeds 100 mm Hg, four-hourly recording whilst the patient is awake becomes desirable. The fetal heart rate (noting rhythm and volume also) is recorded twice daily at least. The doctor will try to assess the fetal growth. Special investigation of oestriol urinary excretion can be useful.

The obstetrician's aim is to prolong the pregnancy whilst the fetus is still growing, and there is no severe maternal deterioration. After 37 weeks gestation, it may be wise to induce labour. Rest in bed probably improves placental blood flow. Only about 3 per cent of patients who are admitted to hospital will improve sufficiently for discharge home. Many remain in status quo—a few degenerate. After 36 weeks gestation, surgical induction of labour is indicated; in severe cases, occasionally after the 34th week. Occasionally in the earlier cases the cervical os is too tight for induction and a Caesarean Section becomes necessary. Even in mild cases of toxaemia, the pregnancy should not be allowed to continue after term. An imperfect placenta with postmaturity can cause fatal fetal anoxia. Drugs are available to reduce a patient's blood pressure (hypotensive) and to increase the output of urine (diuretics), but modern opinion condemns their use as they tend to mask valuable signs without improving placental function. After surgical induction of labour, a toxaemic patient must be observed closely during labour in case her condition worsens or the fetus becomes distressed. A doctor will usually be present during the second stage. The patient must be discouraged from pushing. Facilities for resuscitating an asphyxiated, possibly abnormally small, baby must be available. Oxytoxic drugs cause a vascular spasm and in cases of toxaemia tend to raise the maternal blood pressure. Consequently these drugs should only be used in exceptional cases during or immediately after the third stage. When such drugs are given, frequent maternal blood pressure recordings should be made. Even with a normal delivery, a vascular spasm may occur immediately after delivery, raising the maternal blood pressure, a vasopressin substance being released from the placenta. Therefore patients with pre-eclampsia must be observed closely for at least 48 hours from the time of delivery. After delivery, even in severe cases, the signs of toxaemia retrogress rapidly. Within 5 days protein will usually disappear: the blood pressure falls more gradually. Four per cent may remain permanently hypertensive. In subsequent pregnancies, pre-eclampsia will occur in about 40 per cent (i.e. less than half). The baby, apart from a low birth weight, appears normal and with care should develop normally.

(2) Hypertensive toxaemia

In this case the patient commences pregnancy with a raised BP (over 130/80 mm Hg). All such patients should be booked for a hospital delivery. If overweight, the doctor will advise a restricted carbohydrate diet. In severe cases (diastolic over 100 mm Hg) the doctor may admit the patient for investigation. The femoral pulses will be palpated to exclude a coarctation of the aorta. The patient's past medical history will be investigated, and enquiries made about family history of hypertension. If, in spite of rest, the diastolic blood pressure is maintained above 100 mm Hg, hypotensive drugs are sometimes prescribed. These, however, do not help placental function.

With hypertension miscarriages, premature labours and antepartum haemorrhages are common. As pregnancy advances, other signs of toxaemia commonly appear and the patient may develop eclampsia. Early induction of labour may be indicated. Hypertensive patients should limit their pregnancies. Family planning and sometimes sterilisation is indicated.

(3) Nephritic Toxaemia

At her first antenatal examination, the patient may give a history of previous nephritis or pyelonephritis. Protein is present in the urine. The patient requires full medical examination and renal function tests. Because pregnancy necessitates extra work by the kidneys, poor function (less than 50 per cent) may require a therapeutic abortion. Poorly functioning kidneys will seldom permit a living baby. As pregnancy advances, the amount of protein in the urine increases and the blood pressure tends to rise. Oedema may occur. If pregnancy is allowed to continue, medical supervision is essential—with excretion of protein the serum proteins may diminish and anaemia is common. Generally labour will be terminated by surgical induction at the 36–37th week. In cases of nephritic toxaemia, the placenta is usually infarcted.

(4) Acute Yellow Atrophy of the Liver

In fatal cases of toxaemia the liver shows signs of atrophy and the patient is frequently jaundiced. A typical case of atrophy, however, may be due to a virus hepatitis or follow the administration of drugs toxic to the liver. The classical picture is that of a patient who vomits late in pregnancy and becomes jaundiced. The disease can be fatal within a few days. Vomiting, especially late in pregnancy, must be treated seriously. Bile in the urine is a serious sign. Induction of labour and delivery is the only cure. Any acidosis should be treated by intravenous glucose. Pregnant women should avoid contact with known cases of infectious hepatitis, and drugs known to be toxic to the liver must not be prescribed.

ECLAMPSIA

Eclampsia is manifested by the occurrence of fits in a patient showing signs of toxaemia.

Eclampsia may occur antenatally, but rarely before the 36th week; during labour, usually towards the end of the first stage; or after delivery within 48 hours. Sometimes a family history of eclampsia can be obtained. Each eclamptic fit resembles an epileptic fit, i.e. a short aura, clonic contractions and twitching followed by a convulsion and ending with coma. Fits may recur at short intervals. Nearly always warning signs are present so that eclampsia is largely preventable. Warning signs are diminished urinary output, rising blood pressure and increased proteinuria. Before a patient has a fit she will, as a rule, complain of a severe temporal headache, possibly blurred vision and epigastric pain. The latter may cause vomiting and in such patients the liver may feel tender.

Management

Eclampsia can be fatal. The more numerous the fits, the worse is the prognosis. Death may occur due to liver or renal failure. In addition there is a high fetal mortality rate. Although midwives will seldom see a case of eclampsia (when antenatal care has been adequate), they must understand how to care for an eclamptic patient. Urgent medical aid must be obtained. The patient must be under constant observation. Adequate indirect lighting is needed in order to observe the patient's colour and to make nursing procedures easy. During a fit the patient is liable to bite her tongue and to become cyanosed. A suitable mouth gag should prevent the former, and oxygen must be available. Sudden noise can precipitate a fit, therefore quietness is important. Medical treatment for eclampsia is constantly changing. Usually heavy sedation is necessary to prevent further fits and doctors are constantly seeking good sedative drugs which have a low toxic action on vital organs. Hypotensive drugs have also had their vogue. Attempts are made to improve renal excretion and to protect the liver. Intravenous glucose is helpful.

If eclampsia occurs prior to labour, the fits must first be controlled, then the doctor will usually induce labour surgically with the minimum of disturbance to the patient. When the patient is in labour a general anaesthetic will control the fits and when the cervix is fully dilated the doctor can hasten a vaginal delivery. *Postpartum eclampsia* has the worst prognosis and the fits may be difficult to control. In every case of eclampsia good nursing is imperative. The patient must be under constant supervision. Careful records must be kept regarding her general condition, i.e. colour, pulse and blood pressure taken about 2 hourly. Every fit must be recorded stating the duration and the condition of the patient afterwards. All medical treatment must be recorded. Usually, the doctor will suggest the insertion of a self-retaining bladder catheter. The quantity of urine may be small but samples should be tested 8–12 hourly. Nothing must be given by mouth because of the danger of vomitus being inhaled. If the urinary output remains poor after delivery, blood analysis becomes essential, and occasionally the patient may require the use of an artificial kidney. With adequate antenatal care a midwife should not encounter a case of eclampsia in a patient's home. If this should arise, urgent medical aid can be supplemented by 'the obstetric flying squad'. Once the fits are controlled, the patient should be sent to hospital with a doctor in attendance. Patients who survive, usually recover completely and only about 40 per cent develop toxaemia during a subsequent pregnancy. Recurrent eclampsia is extremely rare.

ANTEPARTUM HAEMORRHAGE (APH)

Antepartum haemorrhage is defined as vaginal bleeding occurring after 28 weeks gestation and before the baby is born. However, bleeding during the actual labour prior to the third stage, is sometimes termed *intrapartum haemorrhage*. APH is usually from the placental site. If the placenta is normally situated in the upper uterine segment, the bleeding is termed 'accidental'. If it is partially or totally in the lower uterine segment, the term *'placenta praevia'* is used. Rare causes of APH are abnormal cervical lesions, e.g. polyp, carcinoma or a haemorrhagic erosion. Very occasionally an abnormal vulval varicose vein will rupture. Occasionally a vasa praevia will rupture when the placenta has a velamentous cord insertion.

Accidental APH is frequently associated with toxaemia and in many instances the signs of toxaemia are exaggerated after bleeding occurs.

Other possible causes include:

(1) A fall or other trauma to the abdomen
(2) An abnormally short cord or one wound around fetal parts
(3) External version
(4) Megaloblastic anaemia
(5) Lack of vitamin C or K
(6) Polyhydramnios after release of excess liquor

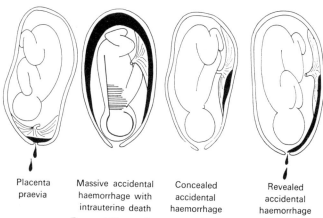

| Placenta praevia | Massive accidental haemorrhage with intrauterine death | Concealed accidental haemorrhage | Revealed accidental haemorrhage |

FIG. 14.6 Types of antepartum haemorrhage

In a number of patients the cause is left undetermined.

Accidental haemorrhage is divided into three types:

(1) Revealed
(2) Concealed
(3) A mixture of 1 and 2

(1) *Revealed APH*

This has to be distinguished from an excessive show. The patient must be admitted to hospital. Blood will be sent for cross-matching in case a transfusion is required. A careful history must be obtained to determine any likely cause. The condition of the fetus must be determined and signs of toxaemia looked for. Further treatment depends mainly upon the period of gestation, the condition of the fetus, and the likely cause.

If gestation exceeds 36 weeks, active treatment is indicated; usually low rupture of the forewaters suffices. This stimulates labour and after the liquor has drained from the uterus the fetus compresses the placenta making further separation difficult. During the subsequent labour, fetal distress must be watched for closely, and after delivery a post-partum haemorrhage (PPH) must be expected and prevented. If the bleeding has been slight and the gestation is less than 36 weeks, close observation in an antenatal unit should be arranged. Once bleeding has ceased, a speculum examination should be done to exclude any lower genital tract cause.

(2) *Concealed APH*

This is serious. The fetus usually dies quickly. The bleeding may begin as a retro-placental clot, but bleeding can be profuse, paralysing the uterus which will enlarge and become inert. The blood can seep through the uterine wall to the peritoneal surface. Although the blood clots within the uterus at first, the maternal circulation soon becomes deprived of fibrinogen and the mother will continue to bleed. Signs of toxaemia are usually present. The patient will soon become shocked and this will affect the blood flow to her kidneys. Subsequently, renal cortical necrosis may develop.

Signs and symptoms. These depend upon the cause and quantity of the bleeding. A retroplacental clot may not affect the patient herself, but the fetal heart may cease. The diagnosis may only be made when the placenta is examined after delivery. A typical case of severe concealed APH presents evidence of shock, a tender excessively large, woody-hard (ligneous) uterus. Protein is present in the urine and occasionally blood and haemoglobin; the urinary output may be scanty. Low fibrinogen levels are usual in the circulating blood. Urgent blood transfusion, sometimes with several pints, is imperative. When the maternal condition improves, the uterine tone will usually recover and some blood is expelled vaginally. When this occurs the forewaters can be ruptured and labour conducted as described under the revealed type of APH. A blood transfusion should be maintained throughout labour. Renal excretion must be closely observed for at least 48 hours after delivery. The third type of accidental haemorrhage is conducted as already described under the revealed type. Very rarely, where there is fetal distress, delivery by Caesarean Section is justified.

PLACENTA PRAEVIA

Four types are described.
(a) *1st Degree*. The placenta is partially in the lower uterine segment but the lower edge is less than 5 cm from the cervix. In the old terminology this was called a lateral placenta praevia.
(b) *2nd Degree*. The placenta reaches the edge of the cervix and the placenta can be felt on a vaginal examination. In the old terminology this was called a marginal placenta praevia.
(c) *3rd Degree*. The placenta covers the cervix when closed, but when the cervix dilates some membrane can also be felt.
(d) *4th Degree*. The placenta completely covers the cervix. Types 3 and 4 were known as central placenta praevia in the old terminology.

The cause of placenta praevia is often said to be unknown. It may occur in any pregnancy but is common in the grand multipara. The logical suggestion is that the fertilised ovum fails to embed in the normal upper uterine segment, almost miscarries but then embeds before reaching the cervix. Placenta praevia does not tend to recur and is not associated with any known uterine abnormality.

Signs and Symptoms. These vary with the degree of placenta praevia. A first degree may only cause a postpartum haemorrhage and be recognised on careful examination of the membranes after the 3rd stage of labour. Other degrees, especially the central type usually give a warning show prior to labour, but more commonly in

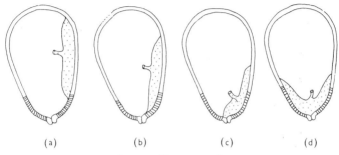

| (a) | (b) | (c) | (d) |

FIG. 14.7 Placenta praevia

the latter weeks of pregnancy—the bleeding is painless. The central type of placenta praevia is frequently associated with an abnormal presentation, e.g. shoulder or a high vertex, because a central placenta praevia prevents normal engagement of the presenting part.

Diagnosis. In types 2, 3 and 4 the placenta can be felt vaginally but this examination may promote further bleeding. Soft tissue X-ray can often show the position of the placenta, especially near term when the placenta contains calcium. Modern sonic apparatus can detect the position of the placenta.

Management. Any bleeding during pregnancy is abnormal. Patients with bleeding must be referred to hospital and admitted. A careful history and clinical examination of the abdomen, urine and blood pressure may suggest placenta praevia. Blood should be taken for cross-matching. Further treatment depends upon the amount of bleeding and period of gestation. Prior to 36 weeks, conservative treatment is best. This entails *strict* bed rest in order that all vaginal loss can be examined. After the 36th week, active treatment depends upon the degree of placenta praevia. In types 1 and 2 low rupture of the membranes can control bleeding. The central types necessitate delivery by Caesarean Section. The low placental site increases the risk of puerperal sepsis. Without conservative treatment many babies die because of prematurity. There is a slight increased risk of a fetal abnormality, presumably because the lower uterine segment is not the optimum site for placental implantation. If blood is inspired into the lower bronchioles a secondary pulmonary collapse can be fatal to the baby. Placenta praevia is frequently associated with a risk of PPH. The placenta may not separate normally and the lower uterine segment has little power of retraction. In the 2nd (marginal) type situated posteriorly, fetal distress may occur during labour because the fetus can compress its own cord. In such cases, shown by X-ray placentography or by fetal distress during labour, a

Caesarean Section delivery may be necessary. Very occasionally bleeding persists after the forewaters have been ruptured and, in a multipara, application of Willetts' forceps to the fetal scalp can control bleeding. A sterile tape is attached to the forceps and a weight, e.g. 8 oz (280 g) is placed at the foot of the bed, so that steady traction is maintained on the fetal head. This old method is only used occasionally. If Willetts' forceps are applied for more than about 8 hours serious scalp infection may occur. Excess traction can promote delivery through an undilated cervix with serious sequelae.

TUMOURS AND PREGNANCY

(1) Fibroids

Cervical fibroids are rare in pregnant women because they tend to cause sterility. Fibroids found during pregnancy are usually extraperitoneal, but they may be intramural. Fibroids tend to degenerate (red degeneration) during pregnancy. This may cause pain, tenderness and a slight pyrexia. Fibroids may cause an abortion

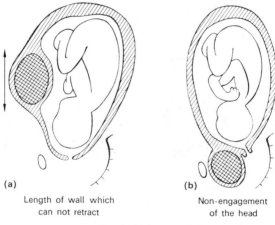

(a)   (b)

Length of wall which   Non-engagement
can not retract   of the head

FIG. 14.8 Fibroids: (a) intramural, (b) cervical

or premature labour. Conservative treatment is best. If pain should occur rest in bed and analgesics are indicated.

During labour, fibroids (especially if intramural) can interfere with normal uterine contractions and prolong the first stage. A postpartum haemorrhage can be severe. During the puerperium the fibroids may become infected and degenerate. It is dangerous to operate during pregnancy and the puerperium because of the increased blood supply to the uterus.

(2) Ovarian Cysts

If diagnosed during the first half of pregnancy the cyst should be removed. Because the cystic ovary may contain the corpus luteum (essential for the maintenance of pregnancy) the operation should be delayed until after the twelfth week, when the placenta has fully developed and can produce ovarian hormones. Ovarian cysts grow rapidly during pregnancy and it is always possible that an ovarian cyst may be malignant. An ovarian cyst can obstruct labour. During the puerperium an ovarian cyst readily twists causing severe pain and an abdominal emergency.

(3) Pelvic Tumours

Bony tumours are rare but would obstruct labour.

(4) Breast Tumours

Any swelling is abnormal and could be malignant. Therefore midwives must be taught how to palpate the mammary glands. The patient should sit and the midwife feels the left breast using her right hand whilst standing on the right side of the patient. For palpation of the right breast the midwife should change sides and use her left hand. The most common swelling is a simple fibroadenoma which feels mobile with no deep attachment. In the puerperium a blocked duct can cause a simple galactosaemia. If the midwife feels any swelling she must obtain medical aid.

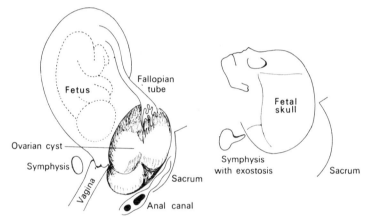

FIG. 14.9 Pelvic tumours

Carcinoma of the breast during pregnancy is very serious, pregnancy activating the lesion. Interruption of the pregnancy may be necessary, but even with this and surgical removal of the tumour, the prognosis is poor. When a tumour has been diagnosed, usually at least a biopsy will be taken or the swelling 'needled'. Occasionally a little blood is excreted through the nipple, more commonly in the puerperium than during pregnancy. Blood may come from a simple duct papilloma but can be an early sign of a breast carcinoma. Malignant cells should be looked for in the breast secretion. Lactation should be suppressed.

POLYHYDRAMNIOS

Polyhydramnios means an excessive accumulation of liquor amnii, greater than 3000 ml. Maternal causes are *Diabetes mellitus* or severe heart disease. Fetal causes are failure of the fetal swallow reflex as occurs in anencephaly, tracheo-oesophageal fistula or an upper intestinal atresia. Polyhydramnios is common in uniovular twins. Severe rhesus immunisation is another cause.

Polyhydramnios is very rare before the 28th week of pregnancy. The onset is usually gradual, but occasionally can be sudden when acute abdominal pain occurs with vomiting and constipation. Diagnosis of polyhydramnios is usually made by abdominal examination, the uterus looking and feeling large for the period of gestation. Fetal parts may be difficult to feel, the fetal heart may be muffled and sometimes a fluid thrill can be elicited. The circumference of the abdomen will increase by more than the usual 2·5 cm per week. The patient may be aware of the rapid increase in the size of her abdomen; she may feel uncomfortable and complain of insomnia.

If a midwife suspects polyhydramnios she should obtain medical aid. The doctor will usually arrange for an X-ray to discover any gross fetal abnormality. If this is found, the patient should be admitted to hospital for induction of labour. In other cases the patient may benefit from rest in hospital. Excess discomfort can be relieved by withdrawing some liquor by abdominal paracentesis: this may have to be repeated.

Pre-eclampsia is a common complication of polyhydramnios. Sometimes polyhydramnios is only appreciated when the patient is in labour. Polyhydramnios can cause a primary uterine inertia, prolonging the first stage. Sometimes excess liquor is only discovered when the membranes rupture; then there is a real risk that a loop of cord will prolapse. A postpartum haemorrhage is likely. The midwife should have obtained medical aid. The baby must have a tube passed into the stomach to exclude a tracheo-oesophageal fistula, before feeding.

OLIGOHYDRAMNIOS

The uterus contains little liquor. The usual causes are a fetal renal abnormality, or poor placental function associated with toxaemia or postmaturity. The uterus will feel small for the period of gestation. During labour fetal distress is common because the fetus will be compressed by each uterine contraction. With renal agenesis only two cord vessels may be present; talipes or congenital dislocation of the hip joints are common.

MULTIPLE PREGNANCY

Twins are relatively common (about 1 in 80 pregnancies); triplets are rare (about 1 in 5000 pregnancies). Quadruplets, quintuplets or more are exceedingly rare. They can occur when an infertile patient receives treatment with human pituitary hormones, unless the dosage is carefully controlled. Midwives are only likely to encounter twins. They tend to be familial. Twins are of two types, uniovular and binovular.

UNIOVULAR (monochorionic) TWINS

One ovum is fertilised by one spermatozoon, the early morula dividing and developing into two fetuses. They are identical in appearance, sex and blood groups. They share one placenta where the circulations communicate. There is only one chorion but each fetus produces a separate amniotic sac.

BINOVULAR (dichorionic) TWINS

The ovary produces two ova simultaneously and each is fertilised by a spermatozoon and develops independently. These twins may be of the same or opposite sexes, their blood groups can differ and their appearances only resemble that of any sibling. Two placentae form with two chorions and two amniotic sacs. The placentae

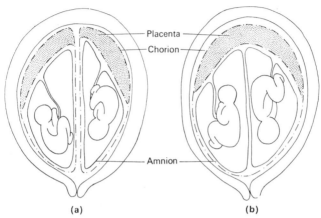

(a)   (b)

FIG. 14.10 Twins: (a) binovular (dichorionic), (b) uniovular (monochorionic)

may be closely adherent. The type of twin can only be determined by careful examination of the placentae after birth.

Diagnosis of twins. The uterus will appear large for the period of gestation. After about the 29th week it may be possible to palpate two fetal heads and extra limbs.

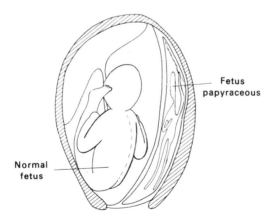

FIG. 14.11 One fetus fails to develop and becomes papyraceous

Theoretically, two fetal hearts can be counted at different rates simultaneously by two observers. One twin may lie posterior to the other and only one head be felt. This will feel relatively small for the size of the uterus.

Complications. Polyhydramnios is common, especially if the twins are uniovular. Anaemia is common, both iron and folic acid deficiency. Pre-eclampsia is common. Occasionally one fetus fails to develop and becomes papyraceous (especially in the uniovular type).

Uniovular twins are occasionally joined together (Siamese). The extra large uterus may cause discomfort and pressure symptoms, interfering with digestion and sleep. Premature labour is common. A first degree placenta praevia is also common.

Management. When a midwife suspects a multiple pregnancy medical aid must be obtained. The diagnosis can be confirmed by X-ray examination. Twins should be delivered in hospital. The patient must have a good diet and obtain extra rest. Complications should be recognised early.

Labour

This is often premature. The optimum length of pregnancy is probably 38 weeks. Postmaturity is associated with fetal asphyxia because a twin placenta may degenerate early. The first stage of labour can be prolonged by uterine inertia. If polyhydramnios is diagnosed some liquor can be released by rupturing the forewaters of the first fetus. Each fetus tends to be smaller than in a single pregnancy, therefore there is more room in a normal pelvis for the cord to prolapse. The most usual presentations are two vertices, but one may be a breech and occasionally the second lies transversely. A doctor should be present for the delivery. During the second stage the first child is born, followed by the second and later the placentae.

Very rarely the twins become locked. This will only occur if the first presents as a breech and the second as a vertex, this head entering the pelvis in front of the first.

Equipment for resuscitation of asphyxiated babies must be available and a competent paediatrician should be present. After the first baby has been born a specimen of cord blood should be obtained for grouping. When the cord is divided the placental end must be securely clamped (in case the twins are uniovular). Some distinguishing mark should be placed on this cord in order that later examination of the placenta can show which portion belonged to each baby. After the first baby has been born uterine contractions usually cease for a period. The position of the second twin must be determined by abdominal examination and the fetal heart checked. Should the lie be oblique an external version is usually possible.

If contractions fail to recommence within about 10 minutes, a vaginal examination should be done; if the presenting part is entering the pelvis the membranes can be ruptured. Contractions usually return; if not, a pitocin (or syntocinon) drip may be given. Occasionally bleeding occurs before the birth of the second twin, indicating usually, that a portion of placenta has separated. If the placental circulations communicate (as in the uniovular type) the second fetus may become anaemic and anoxic. Bleeding necessitates hastening the delivery of the second twin. The cord blood from the second baby should be sent for grouping. After both babies have been born the doctor will usually inject ergometrine 0·5 mg IV, because the large placental site tends to cause a PPH. The placentae should be expelled together. It is important to ensure that the uterus continues to contract well. Ideally, the placentae should be sent to a pathologist for examination and a dye can be injected into the cord blood vessels. This will ascertain whether the twins are uniovular or binovular.

The Puerperium

The extra large uterus will take longer to involute. Involution should be at the usual rate (1·25 cm daily). A mother of twins usually produces adequate milk, but may find difficulty in coping with two babies sucking simultaneously. The babies should change from one breast to the other at alternate feeds in case one sucks better than the other, thus stimulating more milk production.

After leaving hospital the mother of twins requires domestic help. This can be provided by a 'home help'.

TRIPLETS

Triplets occasionally develop from one ovum; more commonly two ova are fertilised and two identical twins and one other baby produced. Rarely, three ova are fertilised by three spermatazoa. Symptoms and complications are the same as for twins but more exaggerated.

During labour all three babies should be born, followed by the placentae.

15 COMPLICATIONS OF LABOUR I: MALPRESENTATIONS

This includes all presentations other than an occipito-anterior.

(1) OCCIPITO-POSTERIOR PRESENTATION

This is either a VROP or VLOP (see page 59).

Diagnosis. On antenatal examination the abdomen appears rather flat. It is difficult to feel the fetal back although it may be felt in one or other flank. The vertex

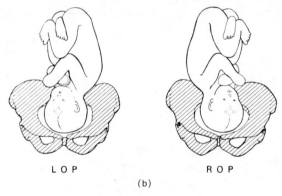

LOP   ROP

(b)

FIG. 15.1 Positions of cephalic presentation: ROP = right occipito-posterior; LOP = left occipito-posterior

usually remains high, even in a primigravida, until labour begins. The fetal heart is usually heard best in the mid-line, although it can sometimes be heard in the flank over the fetal back. There is no antenatal treatment.

Mechanism in Labour

Because the fetal spine tends to be extended by the maternal spine, the fetal head is not fully flexed. The diameter to engage in an oblique diameter of the pelvic brim is usually the occipito-frontal (11·5 cm). This large diameter causes the vertex to remain high until labour begins. Sometimes the subocciptal-bregmatic diameter enters and the head engages before term. During labour there are three possibilities:
(1) If uterine retraction is good the head engages, becomes more flexed so that the occiput reaches the pelvic floor first. It is rotated through three-eighths of a circle to the symphysis pubis and thereafter delivery is normal. If the maternal pelvis is normal this is the usual outcome.
(2) If uterine retraction is poor or the ischial spines are prominent, the fetal head may fail to rotate past the transverse diameter and deep transverse arrest of the head will occur, with the sagittal suture in the transverse diameter.

(3) With a good pelvis the baby can be born in an occipito-posterior position, but this means large fetal diameters emerge and there is tension on the perineum, often resulting in a severe perineal tear.

Management. Fairly frequently, labour fails to commence at term and induction of labour may be required. A midwife must seek medical aid if in a primigravida the fetal head remains high after the 36th week of pregnancy. The midwife should also obtain medical aid whenever the fetal head remains high after labour has begun.

With an occipito-posterior position the first stage of labour tends to be prolonged with poor contractions. The patient should be encouraged, when in bed, to lie on the side opposite to the fetal back. There is a greater risk of fetal distress than in VLOA because extension of the fetal head causes extra strain on the tentoria. The fetal heart must be auscultated at frequent intervals, preferably hourly during the day and when the patient wakens at night. The patient may complain of severe backache. Gentle massage of the back can help. If the pain is severe the doctor may inject a local anaesthetic into the paracervical tissues; alternatively an epidural anaesthetic can be given. With this, pain relief is dramatic and the cervix will usually dilate quite rapidly. If the occiput remains posterior, the sinciput tends to compress the urethra, making spontaneous micturition difficult. A catheter may have to be passed. The urine should be tested for acetone.

If the first stage is prolonged, medical aid must be sought. Sometimes delivery by Caesarean Section will be performed. If the second stage becomes abnormal, i.e. the fetal head fails to advance, the doctor must be called. The doctor can hasten the delivery by applying forceps after rotating the occiput anteriorly, sometimes using Kielland forceps. An alternative method of delivery is by the ventouse vacuum extractor. Usually the doctor performs these operations under local anaesthesia but sometimes a general anaesthetic is advisable. If the fetal head is advancing with the occiput posterior, the midwife may need to perform an episiotomy to prevent a severe perineal laceration.

(2) FACE PRESENTATION

There are four possible positions determined by the position of the chin or mentum:

Left mento-anterior (LMA)
Right mento-anterior (RMA)
Left mento-posterior (LMP)
Right mento-posterior (RMP)

If the chin is anterior a small diameter (the submento-bregmatic, approximately 9·5 cm) will engage in an oblique diameter of the pelvic brim. With descent the chin reaches the pelvic floor and is rotated anteriorly to the symphysis pubis. Thereafter the chin emerges, followed by the face and there should be no anxiety. With a mento-posterior, provided full extension is maintained and the chin reaches the pelvic floor first, a long (three-eighths of a circle) rotation is possible, bringing the chin under the symphysis pubis. Unfortunately the chin can remain posterior and this makes a normal delivery impossible.

Diagnosis. This is difficult during pregnancy. Theoretically one should feel the occiput on the same side as the fetal back. Usually the diagnosis is made during

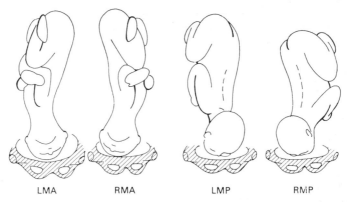

LMA   RMA   LMP   RMP

FIG. 15.2 Varieties of face presentation

labour by feeling the chin, mouth and orbital ridges on a vaginal examination. Many face presentations are due to a fetal abnormality, e.g. anencephaly. A face will present if there is a fetal neck tumour such as a goitre. Some are due to excess activity of the fetal extensor muscles. A few face presentations are due to a pelvic deformity.

Management. If a midwife recognises a face presentation during labour she must obtain medical aid. Provided the chin is anterior, a normal delivery can be anticipated. It is wise, however, to perform an episiotomy in a primigravida at term because there will be extra tension on the perineum.

If the chin is posterior a Caesarean Section may be advisable. Occasionally, the doctor can rotate the chin anteriorly and deliver the fetus with forceps, provided the second stage of labour has been reached. An abnormal fetus (e.g. anencephaly) should have been diagnosed antenatally because of associated polyhydramnios. The baby delivered as a face will have a caput causing swelling over the face and eyes. The appearance can upset the mother and she will require reassurance. The baby is usually cot nursed for 24 hours. Thereafter the baby, as a rule, sucks

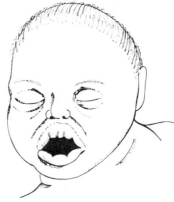

FIG. 15.3 Oedema of a baby's face following delivery of a face presentation

without difficulty. Although the fetal diameters with a face presentation are relatively small, the facial bones are unable to mould.

(3) BREECH PRESENTATION

The fetal head is in the uterine fundus and the lower pole of the fetus presents. The following varieties occur:

(1) *Fully flexed breech.* The legs and thighs flexed, the heels being beside the buttocks.
(2) *Extended legs* (frank breech). The buttocks present and the legs are extended with the feet close to the vertex. This makes diagnosis difficult on abdominal examination.
(3) *Footling presentation.*
(4) *Knee presentation.* This is relatively rare.
(5) *Other possible presentations.* Each fetal leg can assume a different position, i.e. one may be flexed, the other extended.

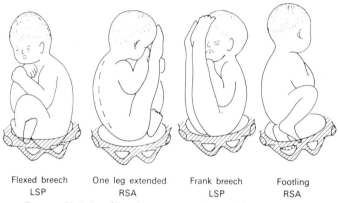

Flexed breech   One leg extended   Frank breech   Footling
LSP   RSA   LSP   RSA

FIG. 15.4 Varieties of breech presentation (LSP = left sacro-posterior, RSA = right sacro-anterior)

Causes of Breech Presentation

(1) Pelvic deformity, i.e. small brim, placenta praevia or an ovarian tumour which makes it difficult for the vertex to engage.
(2) The early occurrence of labour, i.e. prior to the 34th week a breech presentation is common because it is only during the later weeks of pregnancy that the vertex normally descends.
(3) Sometimes the length of umbilical cord and placental site makes a breech presentation the optimum position for the fetus.

Diagnosis during pregnancy. A flexed breech should be readily recognised on abdominal examination. The presenting part feels broad, irregular and softer than a vertex. The fetal head can be ballotted at the fundus. The fetal heart will be heard best above the umbilicus. A breech with extended legs can be difficult to recognise. Frequently the buttocks descend out of abdominal reach and the head will not move easily because of the position of the feet. The fetal heart should still be heard best above the umbilicus. The usual differential diagnosis will be from an occipito-posterior position.

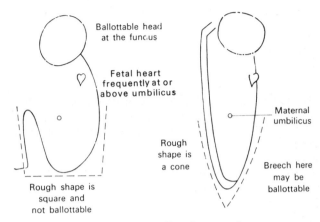

Ballottable head
at the fundus

Fetal heart
frequently at or
above umbilicus

Maternal
umbilicus

Rough
shape is
a cone

Breech here
may be
ballottable

Rough shape is
square and
not ballottable

FIG. 15.5 Palpation of breech presentation

Mechanism in Labour

There are four possible breech positions:

    BLSA—Breech left sacro-anterior
    BRSA—Breech right sacro-anterior
    BRSP—Breech right sacro-posterior
    BLSP—Breech left sacro-posterior

The breech (bi-ischial or bitrochanteric diameter 10 cm) engages in an oblique diameter of the pelvic brim (12·0 cm). Descent occurs during labour and the anterior buttock should reach the pelvic floor first, then one-eighth of a circle internal rotation brings the anterior buttock under the symphysis pubis. This buttock emerges first, followed by the posterior. The shoulders engage in the same diameters and the anterior one should be born first. The head then engages in the opposite oblique diameter of the pelvic brim. The head is slightly deflexed (sub-occipito-frontal diameter 10 cm) and there is no time for moulding. The occiput should descend first and be rotated under the symphysis pubis and be born first.

Danger of a Breech Delivery

(1) The umbilical cord and the fetus are in the pelvis at the same time. There is a real risk of cord compression and fetal asphyxia.

(2) The head has no time to mould.

(3) Rapid exit of the fetal head can promote a tentorial tear and intracranial haemorrhage.

(4) The breech, especially if flexed or when a foot presents, leaves waste space in the pelvis. The umbilical cord can prolapse after the membranes have ruptured. In addition the umbilical cord insertion is nearer the breech than the vertex.

(5) As the largest part of the fetus (the head) comes last there is no possibility of clinically comparing the size of the fetal head with the size of the pelvic brim, which is the best way of diagnosing disproportion.

(6) With a footling presentation it is easy for the foot to pass through the cervical os

before full dilatation. When the foot reaches the perineum the patient will instinctively tend to bear down.

(7) Wrongful handling of the baby's limbs or body during delivery can create fatal injuries.

Management. It is imperative to recognise a breech presentation during pregnancy. The midwife must refer the patient to a doctor in time for treatment. Spontaneous version is preferable to any doctor's manipulation. How long one waits for this possibility depends upon the doctor in charge. In a primigravida 34 weeks seems reasonable, in a normal multipara 36 weeks. The doctor must think of the possible cause for the breech presentation and usually will attempt to perform an external version.

External version. The patient should have emptied her bladder and be relaxed on a couch. The doctor gently eases the buttocks (by abdominal manipulation) out of the pelvis into an iliac fossa. It is helpful if an assistant keeps them there. The doctor then grasps the fetal head and maintaining flexion of the fetal back turns the head towards the pelvis. Only gentle force is justified. Immediately after external version the fetal heart must be auscultated in case the cord has become twisted.

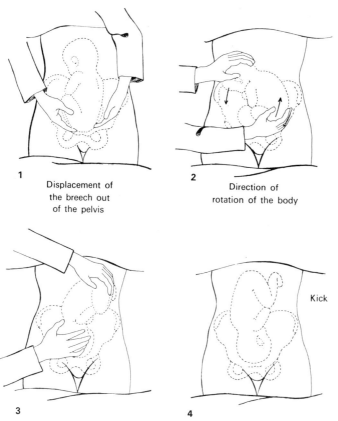

1   Displacement of
the breech out
of the pelvis

2   Direction of
rotation of the body

3

4   Kick

FIG 15.6 External cephalic version

Nowadays external version under general anaesthesia is rarely performed. External version is not always possible, especially when the legs are extended and therefore some babies will be delivered breech first. These deliveries must always be in hospital where a consultant obstetrician is in charge. The maternal pelvis must be carefully assessed prior to labour, sometimes by X-ray measurement (pelvimetry). For the best results the fetus must not be too large and labour will sometimes be induced.

Labour

Diagnosis. If a flexed breech is not recognised on abdominal palpation, a rectal or vaginal examination shows the absence of the vertex. The differential diagnosis is from a face presentation.

A frank breech is more difficult, but with this no suture lines can be felt. A foot must be differentiated from a hand. The foot is typified by the right-angled calcaneus.

Management. The midwife must send for medical aid whenever an abnormal presentation, e.g. breech, is recognised in labour. Whenever possible the patient should be transferred to hospital for delivery. If the delivery appears to be imminent the midwife may have to do her best, the general practitioner may take over or call a consultant obstetrician, occasionally via the 'flying squad'.

Delivery

First stage. As the membranes should remain intact until the end of the first stage to lessen the risks of a prolapsed cord, it may be wise to keep the patient in bed. Sometimes the first stage is prolonged and a Caesarean Section delivery may be performed.

Second stage. As soon as the patient appears to have reached the second stage of labour, medical aid must be called. The doctor will perform a vaginal examination to ensure that the cervix is fully dilated; only then may the patient be permitted to bear down. When the buttocks begin to distend the perineum, the patient must be

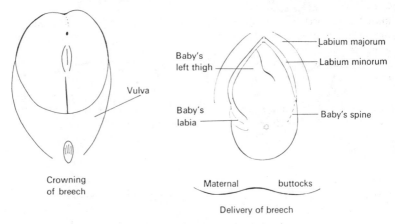

FIG. 15·7 Breech delivery

carefully positioned. Her buttocks must be at the edge of the bed and preferably in the lithotomy position. The doctor will perform a pudendal nerve block with local anaesthesia and usually an episiotomy. The buttocks should descend and be born, the anterior first. The trunk follows and the pulsation in the umbilical cord vessels gives a good guide to the condition of the fetus. The body must be able to hang down as this promotes flexion of the fetal shoulders and head. This explains the importance of correct positioning of the patient. If the pulsation of the cord vessels feels satisfactory, one can await a spontaneous birth of the shoulders. It is important to ensure that the cord is not pulled tight. If the arms are flexed (as is normal) the scapulae can be seen to be close together.

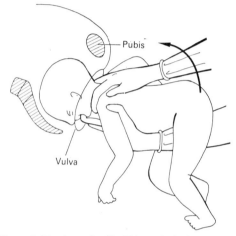

FIG. 15.8 Mauriceau–Smellie–Veit method of delivery of the after-coming head

After the shoulders are born, gentle supra-pubic pressure aids engagement of the head. For delivery of the head, the simplest method is as described by Mauriceau-Smellie-Veit (see Fig. 15.8). The second and fourth fingers of the right hand should grasp the fetal neck, with the third finger on the occiput to maintain flexion. The opposite index finger is in the fetal mouth. If rotation is not complete, this can be achieved. No undue traction on the fetal neck is justified—otherwise serious trauma may arise. If the head fails to advance easily, the doctor may apply forceps to the head and by this means extract the head. Once the fetal mouth has reached the vulva, mucus can be extracted and a slow delivery of the head ensured. All facilities for resuscitation of a possibly asphyxiated baby must be at hand. It is usual to care for a breech born baby in its cot for the first 24–48 hours, watching closely for any signs of cerebral irritation.

Complications

(1) The first stage may be prolonged because of slow cervical dilatation and the presenting part may remain high. The usual treatment will be by a Caesarean Section delivery. Usually the cause is some degree of disproportion.

(2) If the buttocks are slow to descend during the second stage, either there is a

degree of disproportion when Caesarean Section becomes necessary, or the contractions are poor when a pitocin (or syntocinon) infusion will help. If the soft parts are unduly tight, an episiotomy may be necessary. The birth of the shoulders

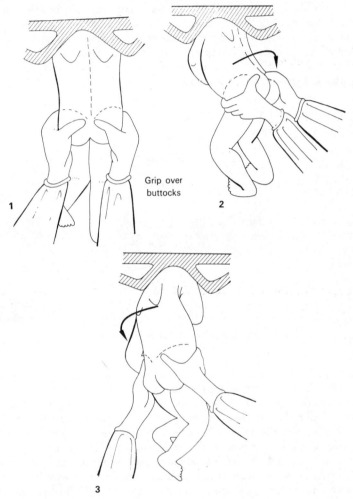

Grip over
buttocks

FIG. 15.9 Løvset's manoeuvre in breech delivery

can be delayed if the arms are extended or dorsi-flexed. Extension is rare provided the buttocks have been born spontaneously and the trunk allowed to hang down. Assistance may be needed, especially if pulsation of the cord becomes slow. Løvset's manoeuvre may be required (see Fig. 15.9).

(3) Delayed delivery of the head may be because the head is too large for the pelvis, or because the occiput has failed to rotate under the symphysis pubis, or because the cervix is incompletely dilated. Disproportion should have been recognised in time

for delivery by Caesarean Section. Rotation of the occiput is achieved by using the Mauriceau-Smellie-Veit manipulation. Delivery through an undilated cervix must be prevented, by encouraging the patient to inhale gas and oxygen until full dilatation of the cervix has been checked by a vaginal examination. In rare cases the doctor may have to incise the cervix, thereafter delivering the fetal head with forceps.

Occasionally a breech delivery is rapid. The fetus may have to be supported and the only safe parts to grasp are the feet or pelvis.

(4) BROW PRESENTATION

When a brow presents the large mento-vertical diameter (13·5 cm) is unable to enter a normal pelvic brim. A brow is difficult to recognise on abdominal palpation but the head will be high.

During labour, occasionally a brow is recognised by feeling the anterior fontanelle and the orbital ridges on vaginal examination. Usually delivery will have to be by Caesarean Section. Occasionally, more often in a multipara with a large pelvis, a brow is recognised in the pelvis, presumably having entered the pelvis as a face presentation. If the cervix becomes fully dilated, a vaginal delivery can be effected by extending the head into a face presentation if the chin is anterior, or flexing the head to an occipito-anterior position if the chin is posterior. It is easier to extend the fetal head. After correction into either of these positions, forceps can be applied and the fetus delivered.

(5) TRANSVERSE OR OBLIQUE LIE (Shoulder presentation)

It is rare for the fetus to lie in the direct transverse axis of the uterus; usually the fetal head is in one or other iliac fossa and the fetal back is either anterior or posterior.

Causes include pelvic brim disproportion, placenta praevia, pelvic tumours, poly-hydramnios or a lax uterus (usually in a grand multipara) or the second twin.

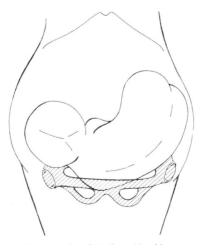

FIG. 15.10 Transverse lie of the fetus (shoulder presentation)

Diagnosis. During pregnancy the abdomen looks wider than normal. The fetal head can be felt in an iliac fossa. During labour frequent uterine contractions can make the diagnosis difficult. A rectal or vaginal examination shows that the presentation is abnormal, no firm presenting part being felt. If the membranes have ruptured, ribs may be felt or an arm; the hand may have passed through the cervix into the vagina. The hand must be distinguished from a foot by the absence of the right angled heel.

Early diagnosis is essential, because it is impossible for the fetus to be born in this position. Labour is dangerous for both mother and baby. The lower uterine segment becomes overstretched and may rupture. The umbilical cord can prolapse and pressure on the fetal chest will cause shock.

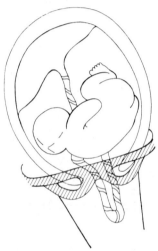

FIG. 15.11 Cord prolapse

Management. If a midwife suspects an oblique lie after the 36th week of pregnancy, medical aid must be sought. The patient should be referred to a maternity hospital. The probable cause will be diagnosed. Should the lie persist after 38 weeks, the patient will be admitted to hospital. Sometimes the fetus will turn spontaneously into a vertex or breech presentation. At the onset of labour, or sometimes when pregnancy has become prolonged, the doctor will push the fetal head gently from an iliac fossa into the pelvic brim and rupture the membranes. Once liquor has drained, the fetus should remain in the longitudinal position and labour will progress.

Treatment in advanced labour is difficult, especially after the membranes have ruptured. Delivery by Caesarean Section is usually necessary. The alternative, internal version, can be difficult and may even precipitate rupture of the lower uterine segment. Internal version requires a general anaesthetic. The hand or shoulder has to be pushed up and the fetal foot brought down through the cervix into the vagina. During this manipulation the cord may be twisted and cause fetal asphyxia. Nowadays internal version is seldom done unless the cervix is fully dilated and the fetus can be delivered immediately by breech extraction.

16 COMPLICATIONS OF LABOUR II: UTERINE AND PELVIC ABNORMALITIES

ABNORMAL UTERINE ACTION

(1) During labour uterine contractions and therefore retraction can be infrequent and weak from the onset. This is termed *primary uterine inertia* (sluggish uterus).

(2) Labour may commence normally but before the delivery has been completed the contractions diminish and may even cease. This is *secondary uterine inertia* (exhausted uterus).

(3) Sometimes contractions are strong during labour but the cervix fails to dilate. This is due to *incoordination* or to a cervical abnormality.

(4) If contractions are unduly strong, labour can be precipitate. If any obstruction is present a pathological *retraction ring* forms between the upper active and the lower passive uterine segment (Bandl's ring).

(5) Occasionally a *constriction ring* develops within the uterus, usually when the uterus has been stimulated by artificial means (manually or by drugs such as pitocin).

(1) Primary Uterine Inertia

Usually insufficient pituitary oxytoxic hormone (pitocin) is produced. Consequently the patient may fail to go into labour at term. This is most common in a primigravida but may occur in a grand multipara. Abnormal presentations can be a cause, e.g. occipito-posterior or breech or when the presenting part remains high. In such cases inertia may result from lack of normal pressure on the cervix. Over-distension of the uterus, as occurs in a multiple pregnancy, or polyhydramnios, can cause inertia.

In a typical case of primary inertia the patient reports because she thinks that labour has begun. Painful contractions are felt but after some hours diminish or pass off. With poor contractions the first stage is prolonged. There should be no fetal distress. Maternal distress is only psychological. If the first stage is prolonged (over 24 hours) the midwife must seek medical aid. After excluding disproportion the doctor may suggest simple stimulation such as an enema and a hot bath. If the membranes are intact the doctor may rupture them and so stimulate contractions. If these methods fail, an intravenous pitocin (or syntocinon) drip may be given by the doctor. A few doctors give pitocin by the buccal route. Whenever pitocin (or synthetic syntocinon) is used the patient must be watched very closely. This artificial stimulation can cause excessively strong uterine contractions leading to fetal distress and occasionally the uterus ruptures. Close observation means taking and recording the fetal heart hourly (when the patient is awake). At the same time the abdomen is palpated to note the frequency and duration of each contraction. The maternal pulse is taken. A midwife should be in constant attendance. The usual dose of pitocin used is one unit per hour given in 5 per cent dextrose. The dose can be doubled if the former proves ineffective. Occasionally higher dosage is required. The drip should be continued until the end of the third stage of labour but the rate at which the drip is running may have to be varied according to the strength and frequency of the contractions. A more modern, less painful labour can be achieved by the use of prostaglandin (prostin E$_2$) but the optimum dosage in tablets has still to be worked out.

If analgesic drugs such as pethidine are given before labour is well established and the cervix dilating, contractions will diminish or even cease. Midwives must prevent this.

(2) Secondary Uterine Inertia

This can only be recognised after the patient has been in labour for some time. Instead of the contractions becoming more frequent and sustained, the contractions diminish and occasionally cease. During the first stage disproportion is the usual cause. In the second stage disproportion may again be the cause, but inertia can occur if the patient becomes exhausted from lack of sleep or early very strong contractions. In the third stage inertia will cause delay or haemorrhage. Midwives must recognise secondary inertia and obtain medical aid. The doctor will deliver the baby if possible before the contractions cease. The third stage complications are dealt with under postpartum haemorrhage (see Chapter 17).

(3) Incoordinate Uterine Action

In this condition the cervix is slow to dilate despite apparently good uterine contractions. Occasionally the cervix is abnormal, either congenitally or due to fibrosis caused by a previous cervical tear or operation. O'Driscoll has suggested that although the uterus may appear to be contracting well the normal pitocin stimulation is lacking, possibly because the two halves of the upper uterine segment are not working in unison. The cervix often feels tight and the external cervical os posterior. Frequently the fetus is in an occipito-posterior position. A frightened patient may stimulate the circular muscles above the cervix to contract but adequate preparation for labour should avoid this.

Incoordinate uterine action causes severe pain and fetal distress. It is most common in a first labour. For years obstetricians have tried different relaxant drugs with variable success. The injection of a local anaesthetic into the parametrium above the cervix (paracervical block) has been advocated. This injection will relieve the pain for a time but the injection has to be repeated and the cervix does not always dilate. A caudal or epidural block anaesthetic is sometimes effective, but this injection requires the presence of a doctor skilled in its use. Provided disproportion can be excluded the controlled intravenous infusion of pitocin or syntocinon causes the cervix to dilate in many cases, reducing the need for delivery by Caesarean Section. In some cases dihydroergotamine 0·25 mgm IM repeated in 1 hour will effect dilatation provided there is no disproportion.

(4) Retraction Ring

Good midwifery should prevent this occurring. Malpresentations, particularly an oblique lie, must be diagnosed early, also disproportion. If a retraction ring forms, the lower uterine segment is in danger of rupturing. A ruptured uterus causes a very high fetal mortality and is also dangerous to the mother. Immediate blood transfusion (sometimes of many pints) and early laparotomy with removal of the uterus may save the mother's life.

Other causes of uterine rupture include:

(a) Administration of oxytoxic drugs
(b) A previous Caesarean Section scar
(c) Previous injury to the uterus as can occur with curettage
(d) Internal uterine manipulation such as internal version
(e) A difficult forceps delivery, especially when the head has to be rotated.

Before a retraction ring has formed the patient will have had strong contractions and her pulse rate will have risen. Pain is severe. When the uterus ruptures the patient temporarily feels better but soon develops shock because of internal haemorrhage. The fetus usually passes through the uterine hole into the peritoneum and dies. Vaginal bleeding is usually slight.

Sometimes the rupture is less dramatic and must be suspected when a patient becomes shocked, especially if her condition fails to improve after a blood transfusion.

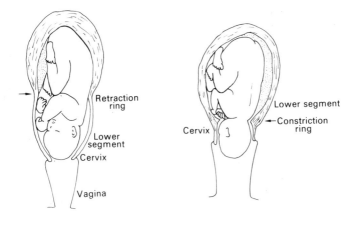

FIG. 16.1. Retraction ring   FIG. 16.2. Constriction ring

(5) Constriction Ring

This ring occurs just above the cervix and can only be felt inside the uterus. This ring is very rare during the first stage of labour. In the second stage it occasionally occurs after prolonged rupture of the membranes, especially if the fetus is dead or after internal manipulation, e.g. internal version. Oxytoxic drugs, particularly an ergot preparation could be responsible, therefore ergot must never be given until the baby has (or in twins, babies have) been completely delivered. By far the most common time for a constriction ring to appear is in the third stage. Previously given ergot may be responsible, or attempting to expel the placenta before separation has occurred.

A midwife should not be confronted with a constriction ring during the second stage of labour, provided she ensures that no ergot preparation is given before the baby is born and the uterus has been palpated to exclude a twin.

A constriction ring must be suspected if, after the fetal head has been born, the shoulders do not appear. In such cases a vaginal examination should detect the ring. Urgent medical aid is required. If the patient inhales a capsule of amyl nitrate the ring may relax, but often deep anaesthesia is required. Steady traction on the fetal head is also necessary. If a constriction ring occurs during the third stage the placenta will be retained. Bleeding is usually minimal. The majority of constriction rings are detected by the doctor only when the placenta is being removed manually because of delay. Generally, the doctor finds that a portion of placenta is still attached at the placental site, i.e. a constriction ring is rare when the placenta has separated.

ABNORMALITIES OF THE PELVIS

The maternal pelvis may develop abnormally or the shape and size can be altered by disease or injury.

Typical developmental abnormalities and their significance to the fetus will be described.

(1) Generally Contracted Pelvis (Justa Minor)

The pelvic shape is normal, but all diameters are smaller than average. Usually, the woman will be small and short. Fortunately such women tend to produce small babies. If the fetal head engages, a vaginal delivery is possible.

(2) Android Pelvis

This pelvis resembles that of the male. The pelvic brim is narrow anteriorly, and the pelvis tends to be deep, with a straight sacrum and prominent ischial spines. The outlet is narrow with a small subpubic angle. If the vertex engages in the occipito-posterior position, the ischial spines make rotation difficult and the narrow outlet may make a vaginal delivery very difficult. Women with an android pelvis are usually tall and they may have some masculine features, e.g. deep voice, excess hair with a male distribution.

(3) Anthropoid Pelvis

This pelvis resembles the shape of that found in anthropoid apes. The antero-posterior diameters of the brim, cavity and outlet are large, but the transverse diameters are small. If the vertex engages in the occipito-posterior position, spontaneous delivery with the occiput posterior usually occurs.

(4) Generally Flat Pelvis (Platypelloid)

All antero-posterior diameters are reduced, but the transverse diameters may be large.

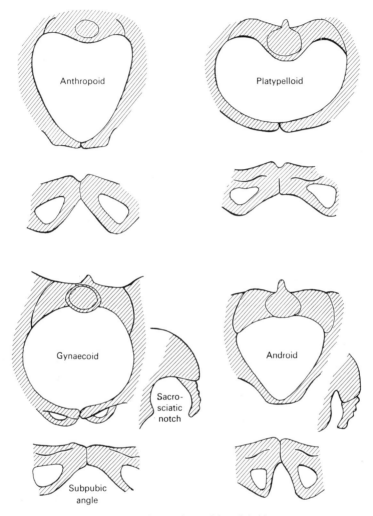

FIG. 16.3 Abnormalities of the pelvis (1)

(5) Gross Abnormalities

Gross abnormalities such as the absence of one sacral ala (Naegele pelvis) or both alae (Robert's pelvis) are very rare. A vaginal delivery of a normal-sized baby is impossible.

The untreated congenitally dislocated hip can cause the pelvis to develop asymmetrically, due to tilting of the pelvis.

(6) Distortion due to other causes

Childhood diseases can alter the shape of the growing pelvis. These include diseases affecting one lower limb, which causes tilting of the pelvis, e.g. poliomyelitis.

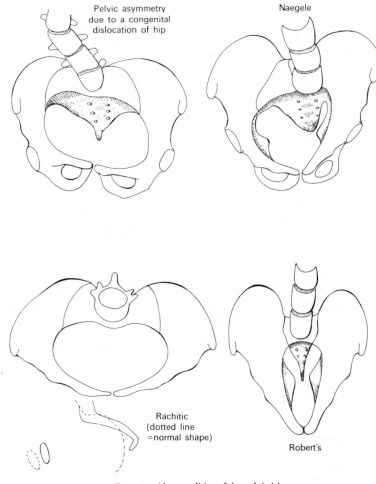

FIG. 16.4 Abnormalities of the pelvis (2)

Spinal diseases, e.g. tuberculosis can change the sacral curve, even if the disease occurs in the upper vertebrae. Diseases of the hip joint may alter the pelvic shape. Rickets can change the shape of the pelvis. When a rachitic child begins to walk, the softened sacral promontory is pushed forward, the iliac crests are pulled back and the subpubic angle of the outlet is enlarged. In consequence, the antero-posterior diameter of the brim is small, but this is the only difficulty the fetus will encounter in passage through the pelvis.

After puberty, the shape of the pelvis is less likely to be altered. Osteomalacia (adult rickets) is rare in this country, but can distort the pelvic bones, making a vaginal delivery difficult. A fractured pelvis (usually caused by road accidents) may form excess callus when healing and this extra bone reduces the size of the pelvis.

It is essential that an abnormal pelvis is detected before a pregnant woman reaches term.

Diagnosis. A midwife should suspect an abnormal pelvis in the following circumstances:

(a) When the patient has had any disease likely to have affected the pelvis.

(b) If the patient is under 5 feet in height.

(c) If there are signs of hirsutism.

(d) If the patient has a limp or evidence of rickets such as bowed legs, bossed forehead or rachitic chest.

(e) If the patient is a multipara and gives a history of previous difficult delivery.

(f) If there is a malpresentation, or if the fetal head fails to engage at the usual time,

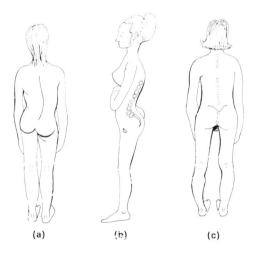

FIG. 16.5 Diseases affecting the shape of the growing pelvis: (a) Kyphosis due to congenital dislocation of the hip, (b) Severe disease (TB) of spine causing marked tilting of pelvis and scoliosis, (c) Rickets. Marked tilting of the pelvis with pot belly and deformity due to poor ossification

i.e. 36 weeks in a primigravida or near term in a multipara. In the latter, a pendulous abdomen may be observed when the patient stands and it is difficult to push the fetal head into the pelvic brim, some overlap being felt.

When a midwife suspects an abnormal pelvis, she must refer the patient to a doctor. An experienced doctor can assess the size and shape of the pelvis by a vaginal examination. Occasionally more accurate measurements are justified. This is done by using X-rays.

Any patient with an abnormal pelvis must be delivered in hospital. The obstetrician will decide on one of three possible lines of treatment.

(1) An elective Caesarean Section

(2) Trial of labour

(3) Induction of labour before term

(1) Elective Caesarean Section

The patient is not allowed to go into labour. She will be admitted to hospital before term. The patient is prepared for a general anaesthetic and an enema is given. A sample of her blood is sent for cross-matching, so that suitable blood is available in case excess bleeding occurs during the operation. Indications for an elective Caesarean Section include a grossly abnormal pelvis (rare), a small pelvis in addition to a malpresentation, such as a breech, and a difficult previous vaginal delivery with a child whose birth weight was not excessive. Sometimes an elective Caesarean Section is performed on an elderly infertile primigravida.

A Caesarean Section, even carefully planned, results in more maternal complications than a reasonably normal vaginal delivery. Apart from early complications, the uterine scar may rupture during a subsequent pregnancy or labour. If a Caesarean Section is done once because of a pelvic abnormality, all later deliveries should also be by this route. Most obstetricians think that three Caesarean Sections should be the maximum number done on one woman.

A vaginal delivery is preferable for the baby. Caesarean Section increases the risk of respiratory distress, so equipment for resuscitation must be available and the presence of an experienced paediatrician is desirable.

(2) Trial of Labour

This is indicated when there is a moderate degree of pelvic contraction in a primigravida who is not elderly or infertile.

Until labour is in progress, it is impossible to foretell how well a fetal head will mould or the degree to which it will flex. Asynclitism can help the head to negotiate the sacral promontory. Strong uterine retraction aids fetal flexion. When good flexion occurs the labour may progress well and lead to a normal delivery. If the head has passed through the pelvic brim and the cervix is fully dilated, the doctor can deliver with forceps provided the pelvic outlet is adequate. Sometimes the fetal head remains above the pelvic brim until the cervix becomes fully dilated, therefore the patient should be allowed to reach this stage before a vaginal delivery has proved impossible.

Sometimes a Caesarean Section is required before this, if fetal or maternal distress arise, or when the first stage becomes prolonged. The patient must be closely observed. The descent of the fetal head can be determined by abdominal palpation. The doctor in charge should be informed when the membranes rupture. After this occurs, if the head remains high, an excessively large caput can form. The patient may need extra sedation as a tightly fitting head can make labour very painful. The patient may find difficulty in emptying her bladder and require to be catheterised. Until the head has engaged there is a risk that the patient will require to be delivered by Caesarean Section, so she must not be given solid food, because of the danger of inhaling vomit if anaesthetised. As a rule, the doctor will perform any necessary rectal or vaginal examinations to assess the cervical dilatation. These should not be undertaken by a midwife during a trial of labour.

(3) Induction of Labour before Term

This would seem to be an excellent way of obtaining a smaller baby, but unfortunately a premature baby's thin skull is susceptible to damage. Induction should not be considered before the 38th week of pregnancy when the pelvis is abnormal.

Labour is induced by rupturing the membranes surgically. There may be a delay before labour commences, allowing the liquor to become infected and this infection can spread to the fetal lungs. If assessment of maturity is not correct the baby could die from immaturity.

COMPLICATIONS OF LABOUR III:
CORD PROLAPSE. POSTPARTUM
HAEMORRHAGE. INDUCTION OF
LABOUR

CORD PRESENTATION AND PROLAPSE

When the umbilical cord is felt either in front of or beside the presenting part before rupture of the membranes, the cord is said to be *presenting*. This is rare. More often the cord will only come down with the gush of liquor amnii when the membranes rupture and the cord is then said to be *prolapsed* (see Fig. 15.11). In such a case, the cord may be felt only on vaginal examination, but sometimes the cord will appear at the vulva.

The causes of presentation and prolapse of the cord are similar, i.e. any malpresentation, disproportion, polyhydramnios, placenta praevia, a relatively small fetus compared with the size of the pelvis, or an abnormally long cord. With prolapse particularly, there is grave risk to the fetus. Pressure on the cord by the presenting part will interfere with the cord circulation and the fetus may die from lack of oxygen. In addition, if the cord emerges at the vulva, the cord vessels may go into spasm and cause fetal asphyxia. There is also a slight risk that the cord may become infected. A midwife will seldom diagnose a presenting cord, but if she does a Caesarean Section is indicated.

When the cord prolapses, urgent treatment is necessary. If the midwife considers that delivery is imminent, the patient must be encouraged to bear down and an episiotomy performed unless the perineum is lax. Otherwise the midwife must send urgently for medical aid and while awaiting this, the patient should be placed in the knee/chest or knee/elbow position or be on her side with the buttocks well raised on pillows; if the cord is on the right side of the pelvis, the patient should lie on the left side and vice versa. The foot of the bed should be raised a few feet, so that the buttocks are at a higher level than the upper abdomen. This position should keep the presenting part out of the pelvic brim. If the cord is outside the vulva, the cord should be covered with a warm sterile towel. If possible, the patient should inhale pure oxygen.

Medical treatment depends on the dilatation of the cervix, the reason for the prolapse of the cord and the condition of the fetus. Before the second stage of labour has been reached, an immediate Caesarean Section will be necessary to save the fetus, the patient remaining tilted until anaesthetised. If the patient is in the second stage of labour, the doctor will hasten delivery by applying forceps or extracting a breech, unless there is some contra-indication to an easy vaginal delivery. Even with the treatment recommended, there is a high fetal mortality, possibly 50 per cent.

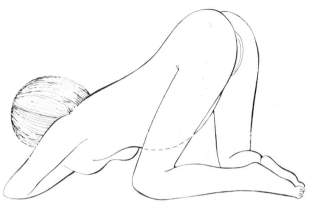

FIG. 17.1 Knee/chest position

POSTPARTUM HAEMORRHAGE (PPH)

This is defined as a blood loss greater than 600 ml, occurring during the third stage of labour, with the delivery of the placenta or after. Known causes include:

(1) *Poor uterine retraction.* This may be due to primary or secondary inertia.

(2) *Partial separation of the placenta* will follow any antepartum haemorrhage or could arise if attempts are made to expel the placenta before this has completely separated.

(3) *Abnormal adherence of part of the placenta.* This is fairly common when there is a succenturiate lobe or where part of the placental site is at a uterine cornu.

(4) *Insertion of the placenta in the lower uterine segment* (placenta praevia).

(5) *Failure of the blood to clot* (*hypofibrinogenaemia*) is a rare cause.

(6) *Bleeding from a tear,* usually of the cervix, but sometimes from the vagina or from an episiotomy.

Prevention is better than cure. Therefore all patients at risk must be delivered in hospital. Such patients include:

(a) Grand multipara (para 4+).

(b) Multiple pregnancies.

(c) Patients with polyhydramnios.

(d) All patients with a previous history of PPH or difficulty in the third stage (because this tends to recur).

(e) All patients who have an antepartum haemorrhage however slight.

(f) All patients with inertia. If inertia arises during labour at home the patient should be transferred to hospital for delivery, if there is time.

Signs of PPH

The occurrence of vaginal bleeding without evidence of placental separation. Occasionally if the uterus is failing to contract, blood accumulates within the uterus and little is expelled. In such cases the uterine fundus will rise but the uterus feels soft.

A patient can become shocked, but the degree depends on the patient's haemo-globin prior to delivery as well as the amount of blood lost. The systolic blood pressure may fall below 100, but it is important to compare the blood pressure with the patient's normal level, because there is a racial variation in 'normal' blood pressure. With shock the patient's pulse rate usually rises, but not always. She becomes pale and her extremities, especially the nose, feel cold and the skin is 'clammy'. Death can ensue.

Treatment

(1) Prophylactic

(a) All patients at risk must be delivered in hospital and should have blood taken and cross-matched so that compatible blood is available if needed.

(b) The doctor usually gives such patients 0·5 mg ergometrine intravenously after the baby has been delivered. The optimum time for the injection is debated by obstetricians. In a doctor's absence the midwife may be asked to give 1 ml synto-metrine IM (this contains 0·5 mg ergometrine and 5 units of synthetic pitocin, i.e. syntocinon). After the oxytoxic drug has been given, attention should be focused upon the uterus. When evidence of placental separation occurs, the placenta should be delivered at once, otherwise a constriction ring can form.

(2) Curative

There should be no bleeding during the third stage until the placenta has separated. Therefore, when the patient begins to bleed the midwife must check for placental separation. If this is not apparent the midwife must send urgently for medical aid. Meanwhile she should stimulate the uterus to contract by massaging the uterus gently. She can give ergometrine 0·5 mg IM (provided oxytoxic drugs have not

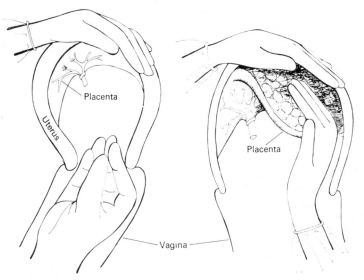

Fig. 17.2 Manual removal of the placenta (abdominal wall not shown)

already been given). Ergometrine usually causes the uterus to contract and reduces the bleeding temporarily. Medical treatment is manual separation and removal of the placenta, usually under general anaesthesia. Therefore the patient must be given nothing by mouth.

Even when patients are selected carefully for home confinement, a PPH may occasionally arise. Unless the midwife can obtain medical aid rapidly, she must call the 'Flying Squad'. An ambulance will bring necessary equipment and group O rhesus negative blood to the patient's home. A senior obstetrician will arrive, sometimes with an additional midwife, and, in many centres, an anaesthetist if required. The 'Flying Squad' is centred at a maternity hospital. Even with good

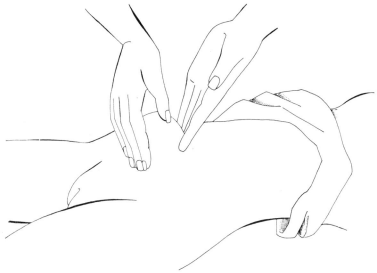

Fig. 17.3 Bimanual compression of uterus

organisation the 'Squad' will take some time to arrive, especially in a busy city when the call arises during peak traffic hours.

Sometimes a PPH arises after the placenta has been expelled. The usual causes are inertia, placenta praevia or a retained placental cotyledon. In these cases the midwife should massage the uterus gently to encourage contraction and repeat 0·5 ergometrine IM. As soon as possible she should send for urgent medical aid.

The placenta must be inspected for any missing cotyledon or placenta praevia; and the placenta must be kept for the doctor to examine. Modified bimanual compression of the uterus will prevent the uterus from filling up with blood. This should be maintained if necessary until the doctor arrives. If the doctor suspects that a placental cotyledon has been retained, the uterus will be explored under a general anaesthetic.

Bleeding from Tears of the Genital Tract

Cervical or high vaginal tears usually cause some bleeding before the baby is born. Sometimes the midwife will know that the patient has been trying to bear down before the cervix is fully dilated. Bleeding from labial or perineal tears, or after an episiotomy, should be obvious on inspection. Any spurting vessel must be secured by a Spencer Wells' forceps. Medical aid is required. The sooner the tear is sutured the better. As a rule, bleeding from tears can be differentiated from bleeding from the placental site. The bleeding from a tear is more constant and the uterus will feel normally contracted.

PPH as described here is primary haemorrhage.

Delayed Primary Haemorrhage

This can occur between 1 hour and 24 hours after delivery. The haemorrhage may appear when the effect of oxytoxic drugs wears off. A full bladder can interfere with normal uterine retraction. A retained placental cotyledon is a likely cause. The midwife must recognise excessive lochial loss and obtain medical aid. Treatment depends upon the cause.

Secondary PPH

Secondary haemorrhage is that occurring more than 24 hours after birth; it usually occurs during the second week or even later. The cause may be a retained placental cotyledon or erosion of the vessels at the placental site by infection. The bleeding can be profuse. The incidence of secondary PPH can be reduced if the midwife delivers the placenta carefully and makes sure that the placenta is complete. The midwife should ensure that the uterus is fully involuted and that the lochia is normal before the patient leaves her care. Ideally, the doctor should check the uterine involution by making a vaginal examination about the 8th–10th day postpartum. A secondary haemorrhage may necessitate a blood transfusion followed by digital exploration of the uterus under anaesthesia. Immediate treatment is the administration of 0·5 mg ergometrine IM. Any infection will require antibiotic therapy.

Obstetric shock

After delivery this is rare without bleeding. A cardinal sign is a fall in blood pressure. A systolic pressure below 100 can be serious. The pulse rate usually rises and the pulse volume becomes poor. The patient's skin, especially the extremities (e.g. nose) feels cold and may be 'clammy'. Sighing respiration can occur in serious cases. Uterine rupture or an inversion of the uterus are possible causes. The midwife must recognise shock and obtain medical aid at once. Meanwhile the foot of the bed should be raised about 18 inches (to maintain cerebral circulation). The patient will feel cold but hot water bottles should not be given, because the skin will burn at relatively low temperatures. Immediate infusion of fluid and blood by the doctor is essential. Prolonged shock can lead to Simmond's disease. This is a distressing condition due to pituitary atrophy. Menstruation ceases permanently and the patient always feels cold.

INDUCTION OF LABOUR

Nature should not be interfered with without good reason, but induction may be desirable to save the patient from serious disease, such as severe toxaemia, or in the interest of the baby.

Indications

(1) *Maternal*

(a) Severe toxaemia.
(b) To prevent a difficult vaginal delivery, as in cases of slight pelvic contraction, or a clinically large fetus.
(c) Fetal abnormality.

(2) *Fetal*

(a) Rhesus immunisation.
(b) Maternal diabetes.
(c) When placental insufficiency is suspected. Occasionally when a twin pregnancy reaches the 38th week.
(d) Toxaemia.
(e) Abnormal presentation such as a breech, where a large baby increases the fetal risk.
(f) Fetal death.

Methods

The most certain way of stimulating labour is surgical, i.e. stretching the cervix, separating and rupturing the membranes. The membranes can be ruptured in front of or above the presenting part. Labour usually commences within 24 hours.

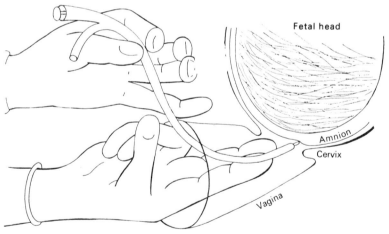

FIG. 17.4 Artificial rupture of membranes by Drew–Smythe catheter

Failing this a pitocin (or synthetic syntocinon) infusion can be given intravenously, aiming at a dosage of 1 unit per hour. If labour does not begin the pitocin dose can be cautiously increased to double or treble the initial dose, but the patient must be watched very carefully in case the contractions become severe, when maternal and fetal distress is likely to occur. An alternative to oxytoxic drugs is to use prostaglandin (prostin E_2) either in tablet form or by the intravenous route. Occasionally when labour fails to start, delivery will be by Caesarean Section.

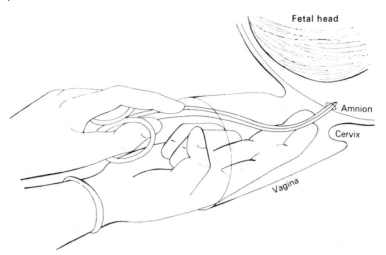

FIG. 17.5 Artificial rupture of membranes by amniotomy forceps

Dangers

There is a risk of introducing infection into the uterus during a surgical induction. If organisms pass into the amniotic cavity they will reach the fetal lungs and cause pneumonia. A surgical induction must only be done under strict aseptic and antiseptic precautions; antiseptic pessaries may be given in advance or the vagina and cervix disinfected at the time. The value of oral antibiotics is under debate. In cases of fetal death a surgical induction is contra-indicated, because dead tissue attracts organisms, such as *Clostridium welchii*, and they can cause a serious uterine infection. For fetal death a pitocin (or syntocinon) infusion can be used, sometimes preceded by oestrogens (usually oral stilboestrol). The dose of pitocin can be increased to 20 units per litre but the patient must be watched closely in case too powerful uterine contractions occur. Some obstetricians give pitocin by the 'buccal' method.

Prior to induction the patient should be given an explanation about the procedure. She will be given an enema to empty the lower bowel, a hot bath and hair will be shaved from the vulval area. Nowadays castor oil is seldom given. During the surgical procedure an inhalant analgesic will help the patient to relax and minimise pain.

Labour has been induced for postmaturity in the belief that placental degeneration would cause fetal distress. Placental insufficiency, it is now realised, does not necessarily occur when the pregnancy is prolonged and may occur before term. It is very important to detect placental insufficiency before the fetus is at serious risk. With placental degeneration the amount of liquor amnii diminishes. This can be suspected on abdominal examination. Reduced liquor causes the patient to lose weight. She may notice a change in the fetal movements.

The quantity of oestriol in a 24 hour specimen of urine varies with the stage of pregnancy, but a falling level indicates placental insufficiency, provided the volume of urine is at least 1000 ml. If the oestriol, after 36 weeks of pregnancy, is less than 10 mg (40 S.I. units) the fetus is at risk.

18 COMPLICATIONS OF THE PUERPERIUM

PUERPERAL PYREXIA

Every patient who develops a temperature of 38° C (100·4° F) within 14 days of delivering a baby, or after a miscarriage, is said to have puerperal fever; and until October 1st 1968 the doctor had to notify the medical officer of health on a special notification form, giving the cause. Puerperal fever has ceased to be a notifiable disease.

A midwife must obtain medical aid if her patient's temperature reaches 100·4° F (38° C) during the early puerperium. The Central Midwives Board also insist that midwives obtain medical aid for any woman whose temperature reaches 37·4° C (99·4° F) on three successive evenings.

Possible causes of Puerperal Pyrexia are:

(1) Genital Tract Infection

The placental site is a raw area and thus the usual site of infection, but a cervical or vaginal, even labial tear, especially unless sutured early, can become infected. Any of the known pathogenic organisms may be responsible. Before the days of sulphonamides, (i.e. before 1935) the haemolytic streptococci were a common cause; later *Staphylococcus aureus*; but nowadays Gram-negative bacilli give most trouble. Infection can reach the genital tract from a focus of infection in the patient (*autogenous*) or an outside souce (*hexogenous*) for instance from unsterile equipment or from the attendant (midwife or doctor).

Prevention. All possible sources of infection in the patient should be treated during the antenatal period, e.g. carious teeth, a vaginal discharge or pyelitis. If the patient has a sore throat or any skin infection when labour commences, the midwife should discover this in order to take necessary precautions, e.g. in hospital the patient will be isolated. During labour every vaginal examination and every manipulation by a doctor (surgical induction, forceps delivery and especially separating the placenta manually) increases the risk of infection, even when strict aseptic and antiseptic precautions are taken. The more normal the labour can be, the less likely is the patient to become infected.

When the vulva is exposed during labour the midwife and doctor should wear adequate masks (covering mouth and nose) to prevent droplet infection. Sanitary pads must be sterile. The patient must not touch her vulval area without disinfecting her hands. Disposable handkerchiefs only should be used by the patient.

During the puerperium, only healthy visitors should come into contact with the patient. In the wards adequate spacing of beds is necessary, also good ventilation; the temperature should not exceed 21° C (70° F) because bacilli thrive at higher temperatures. Damp dusting and vacuum cleaning of the floor surface is necessary. Only boilable blankets should be used. When the patient is allowed to get up for toilet purposes, care must be taken to prevent cross-infection during this procedure.

The patient must be taught how to swab the perineum after defaecation. Frequent changing of sanitary pads is important.

A healthy patient can withstand some infection. It is important to ensure that the patient's haemoglobin reaches 80 per cent (11·5 g) prior to labour. Vitamin A increases her resistance to infection and is available to all pregnant women. She should take one vitamin A and D tablet daily.

Signs and Symptoms of Genital Infection

When infection is limited to the placental site the only signs are offensive lochia and poor uterine involution. Occasionally the temperature rises with a corresponding increase in the pulse rate. Unless infection is recognised and treated early, the pathogenic organisms can pass along the Fallopian tubes causing salpingitis and even reach the peritoneal cavity causing peritonitis. From the placental site the organisms can reach the maternal bloodstream and cause septicaemia. Salpingitis is associated as a rule with a high temperature and pulse rate, and pain in the corresponding iliac fossa. Peritonitis causes abdominal distension and vomiting and sometimes diarrhoea.

In septicaemia, rigors occur and pyaemic abscesses appear in various organs, e.g. heart, lung and kidneys. Rashes are common.

Treatment. Prevention is most important. Midwives must recognise infected lochia and obtain immediate medical aid. The doctor will arrange to send a vaginal swab to a pathological laboratory, so that the organisms can be cultured and their sensitivity tested against various antibiotic drugs. This takes time, so the doctor usually prescribes an antibiotic which will kill the majority of pathogenic organisms, e.g. ampicillin, whilst awaiting the pathologist's report. By the time the report is received, the patient has usually improved, but if she has not, the doctor then knows the best drug to prescribe.

An infected cervical tear will also make the lochia offensive. Infection from a torn cervix can spread along the transverse cervical ligaments to the pelvic fascia. When this occurs the patient complains of backache and her pulse rate is raised more than her temperature. Pelvic cellulitis makes the tissues feel hard and an abscess may ultimately form. The chief danger is thrombosis of the pelvic veins leading to a deep vein thrombosis of the corresponding lower limb. Part of the pelvic thrombus may dislodge and pass via the inferior vena cava to the heart and lung causing a pulmonary embolus which may result in death.

A healthy cervix will not become infected. A midwife should prevent cervical tears by ensuring that her patient does not push down until the second stage of labour. A doctor may tear the cervix during a manipulative delivery: in such cases the cervix must be inspected and any tear sutured at the time.

(2) Pyelonephritis

This is relatively common, especially if pyelitis has occurred antenatally. Failure to empty the bladder completely during labour or during the early puerperium, or the passage of a catheter may lead to infection. As during pregnancy, renal colic is absent because the ureters are still dilated. Rigors are common and a high pyrexia can occur. The diagnosis is usually made by the examination of a midstream specimen of urine. Pyelitis must be suspected in any case of puerperal pyrexia when the genital tract appears to be normal. It is important to recognise and treat pyelitis early, otherwise a chronic pyelonephritis may ensue.

(3) Mastitis

Initially, mastitis is manifested by a high temperature due to a milk protein reaction. The breast shows a small linear area of inflammation in one quadrant. In the initial stage the milk is still sterile. Without early treatment the quadrant soon becomes indurated and tender; later an abscess can develop.

Preventive Treatment. This entails good hygiene and the prevention of cracked nipples. The mother should be taught how to express surplus milk after her baby has sucked. Retained milk is an excellent culture medium for organisms.

Curative Treatment. Mastitis must be treated with antibiotics and the breasts must be emptied, preferably by the baby. Oestrogen therapy should be avoided as this precipitates abscess formation. If a breast abscess develops this will require incision.

Other causes of puerperal pyrexia are chest infections, any erythematous disease or solely a reaction to a difficult delivery.

OTHER PUERPERAL COMPLICATIONS

These include:

(1) Thrombophlebitis

Inflammation and clotting of venous blood is rare during pregnancy but fairly common after delivery. Excess fibrin, released from the involuting uterus, circulates in the blood, and fibrin encourages blood to clot. The lower limb veins are the most vulnerable.

Thrombophlebitis may occur in superficial veins when pain, redness and slight thickening of the vein is obvious. This is not serious unless the inflammation spreads up to the femoral veins. The pain is relieved by applying icthyol and glycerine to the area of inflammation and taking the weight of bedclothes off the limb by using a 'bed cage'.

Deep thrombophlebitis is less obvious and far more serious. There is a real risk of blood clot becoming detached and passing via the inferior vena cava to the heart and lung. A pulmonary embolus can be fatal and is a cause of maternal death. Deep thrombosis may begin in a calf vein or occasionally in a pelvic vein. An early symptom of calf vein thrombosis is pain in the calf, sometimes described by the patient as cramp. If the corresponding foot is dorsiflexed, tension on the affected calf vein causes pain (Homan's sign). Midwives should perform this Homan's test daily during the early puerperium.

Prevention. Early ambulation and active leg movements in bed maintain a good circulation. Anaemic patients are particularly prone to develop thrombosis, therefore anaemia must be prevented, if necessary by giving a blood transfusion when there has been an excess blood loss during delivery.

Treatment. A midwife must obtain immediate medical aid if she suspects any thrombosis. The doctor, after confirming the diagnosis, will usually order anti-coagulant therapy. Intravenous heparin acts rapidly, oral preparations, e.g.

dindevan or warfarin more slowly. Anticoagulant therapy must be controlled by laboratory tests because an overdose can cause bleeding.

Deep vein thrombosis can result in a swollen lower limb. Once this happens, even with anticoagulant therapy, the result is morbidity. The patient in the future complains of a heavy, aching limb, especially premenstrually.

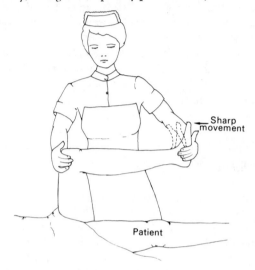

FIG. 18.1 Test for Homan's sign

(2) **Psychosis**

Psychosis is rare during pregnancy, occurring more commonly in the early or late puerperium. Sometimes there is a history of mental instability.

An early sign is insomnia, followed by irrational behaviour. The patient may be depressed or maniacal. She may attempt to commit suicide or infanticide.

If psychosis is recognised early, treatment with tranquillisers may suffice. Some patients will require to be treated in a psychiatric hospital. The ultimate prognosis is usually good but patients improve quicker if the baby can be admitted with the mother.

Psychosis does not always recur after subsequent deliveries.

19 DRUGS

To be of use a drug must act on a specific organ or system of the body and if it is to be safe it must be non-toxic to other cells and tissues. Research chemists are constantly striving to produce more active drugs with the minimum of toxicity. After careful analysis, a drug is generally tested on animals, but before it is released for human consumption, carefully controlled clinical tests on humans are undertaken, usually in hospitals. If proved to be safe the drug can be marketed. However some ill effects may be delayed, and some people may be ultrasensitive. Since January 1964 the Dunlop Committee has required doctors to report any undue drug reaction. As a result of reports the Dunlop Committee may withdraw a drug for further research or remove it permanently from the market. It is imperative that midwives note and report to a doctor when any drug seems to cause a reaction.

Most drugs are absorbed into the blood and excreted by the kidneys, but they may be altered by the liver before excretion. The blood content varies with the dosage and site of administration. The highest levels occur after intravenous administration, the next highest after intramuscular injection and levels are less high after oral administration. Even ointments, e.g. steroids, can accumulate in the blood.

When given by mouth gastric secretions may alter the drug. This alteration can be reduced by suitable coating of tablets. In labour oral drugs take longer than normal to be absorbed, because of a reduction in gastric activity.

In pregnancy most drugs given to the patient will pass through the placenta to the fetus. Fortunately it seems likely that the placenta can alter a drug and save the fetus from an overdose. In the first 12 weeks of pregnancy, when the fetus is developing its vital organs, many drugs are known to be dangerous. This has been shown with thalidomides and any drug may be dangerous. It is important that no drug is given unless it is absolutely essential for the patient's health. During labour analgesic drugs may appear to be desirable but can cause fetal asphyxia. All analgesics must be given with care.

Lactating women secrete drugs in breast milk. During the early puerperium salicylates and sulphonamides should be avoided because these drugs combine with albumin. New-born babies require albumin to combine with bilirubin and prevent jaundice, which could cause kernicterus.

Before a drug is prescribed a doctor should have diagnosed the cause of any complication. If it is infection, the causal organism should be isolated and tested for drug sensitivity. Midwives carry drugs and can give those which they have been taught to use. The drugs carried will depend on their employing authority. Midwives must abide by the Central Midwives rules, e.g. dangerous drugs must be kept under lock and key. All drugs given must be carefully recorded and only correct doses given.

Drugs commonly carried by midwives include:

(1) A simple *sedative* to be given during early labour, e.g. choral hydrate or doriden (glutethimide).

(2) *Analgesics.*

The usual is pethidine. It should be remembered that too early administration during labour can reduce uterine activity and prolong the first stage. If pethidine is given within 4 hours of birth the baby may be asphyxiated. Careful timing is therefore essential. Inhalant analgesics are carried by midwives. They can give nitrous oxide and oxygen by the Entonox machine or else trilene or penthrane. Midwives are trained in the use of inhalant analgesics and receive lectures about them. Reducing the percentage of oxygen inhaled during labour may cause fetal distress, therefore when the patient is inhaling the gas a frequent check on the fetal heart is imperative. When inhalants are administered a second person must be present to look after the machine when the midwife has 'scrubbed up' for the actual delivery. A doctor must certify in writing that the patient is fit for an inhalant analgesic.

(3) *Oxytocic Drugs*

(a) Pitocin or synthetic syntocinon. A midwife can only give this after the drug has been prescribed by a doctor. Pitocin, an extract from the posterior pituitary gland, causes normal uterine contractions of labour. Pitocin may be prescribed to induce labour, usually after the membranes have been ruptured; or to increase uterine contractions where there is inertia. The dosage is easily controlled in an intravenous infusion but some obstetricians use the 'buccal' route. Instead of pitocin (or synthetic syntocinon) prostaglandin (prostin E_2) is now used either in tablet form or intravenously (see pp. 126, 139).

Pitocin is sometimes prescribed for subinvolution during the puerperium. Then it may be given intramuscularly, 2·5 units repeated once after 4 hours.

(b) Preparations of ergot. Ergot contains 3 alkaloids (1) Ergometrine which acts quickly (2) Ergotamine and (3) Ergotoxine, the latter two being slow reactors.

Ergot is marketed in tablet form containing all 3 alkaloids. Oral administration gives a slow but prolonged affect. Two ergot tablets can with advantage be given before the midwife leaves a patient after delivery.

Ergometrine can be given either intravenously by a doctor or intramuscularly by a midwife. The maximum dose is 0·5 mg. Given during or after the third stage of labour, ergometrine stimulates powerful prolonged uterine contractions. Ergometrine must never be given before the baby is born because the prolonged contraction will deprive the fetus of oxygen.

Midwives are now allowed to give ergometrine or syntometrine (syntocin on 5 units and ergometrine 0·5 units) before the placenta has been expelled. In cases of PPH this is most valuable. If ergometrine has been given the midwife must recognise when the placenta has separated and encourage its expulsion before a constriction ring develops. After the third stage ergometrine (or syntometrine) is valuable if the uterus is not contracting well. Excess dosage of ergot can cause a generalised vascular spasm and cases of digital gangrene have been described.

Drugs may alter with keeping. Some become toxic, e.g. sodium bromethol. Some drugs must be kept at cool temperature, e.g. suxamethonium. The type of container can be important. The Dunlop Committee recommend that the name of the drug is recorded on each container.

A midwife should know what drugs, if any, her patient is taking and on admission to hospital the patient should be asked to produce any drugs she has. Drugs in combination can cause dangerous reactions, e.g. monamine oxidase inhibitors (anti-depressants) are dangerous if the patient requires a general anaesthetic. Some foods, e.g. cheese or alcohol, can increase the potency of drugs, e.g. phenobarbitone with alcohol.

HYPNOSIS

Hypnosis has been suggested as an effective method of relieving pain in labour, eliminating the need for analgesics which are potentially dangerous to the fetus. Susceptible patients under hypnosis feel no pain, but not all patients respond to this treatment. Training in this technique, preferably individually but possible in groups, takes time. Normal labour in a relaxed patient should cause little pain and therefore hypnosis can only play a minor part. In abnormal labours hypnosis can be dangerous by masking signs of danger, e.g. a ruptured uterus has been recorded under hypnosis.

Since the reorganisation of the National Health Service all midwives are employed by Area Health Authorities and are responsible to the Divisional Nursing Officers, Midwifery. Midwives may opt to work mainly in hospital or mainly in the community with a varying degree of interchange, depending on local circumstances.

As delivery in hospital is encouraged, many community-based midwives accompany their patients into a G.P. Unit, deliver them and continue their care at home after approximately forty-eight hours.

If a labour is expected to be normal, home delivery is acceptable, but all patients at risk should be delivered in hospital. For a safe home delivery, the basic essentials include running hot and cold water, indoor sanitation and suitable heating and lighting facilities. The patient must never be left in the house during and after delivery without an adult being present. Usually the husband is at home during the night. If he has to work during the day and no other suitable person is available, the patient can employ a 'Home Help' during the early puerperium. Home Helps are women employed by the Social Services Department of the Local Authority who pay their salary. Patients reimburse according to the husband's earnings.

Home Helps receive a short course of lectures and instruction. They attend patients confined at home, ensuring that the house is kept clean, children cared for and meals cooked. Suitable women are in short supply. Many work part-time, some full time from as a rule 9 a.m.–5 p.m.

Antenatal clinics are held in Personal and Child Health Centres with a doctor in attendance, usually a general practitioner (sometimes a public health doctor). At the clinic it is usual for mothercraft and relaxation exercises to be taught. A dentist, employed by the Area Health Authority, examines and treats pregnant women.

CARE OF THE UNMARRIED PREGNANT WOMAN

Pregnancies out of wedlock have become more frequent, possibly because of unsatisfactory sex education and sex prominence in films, stage and television. There is no real evidence that children mature earlier now than in the past.

The unmarried require extra care when pregnant. A young patient may request an abortion without realising the potential dangers. The cervix may be very difficult to dilate without tearing muscular fibres and this can lead to future obstetrical complications. The abortion act was not designed for 'abortion on demand'.

Some young girls want the baby as a 'living doll'. The patient's parents should be encouraged to accept responsibility but this is not always possible. The patient can be admitted into a home for unmarried mothers; the baby can then be fostered or adopted in due course. Medical social workers are employed at most maternity hospitals and advise the unmarried pregnant women.

Homes for unmarried mothers are provided by the Local Authority and Voluntary Organisations. Usually the patient enters the home when she is about 36 weeks pregnant. Some homes are equipped for normal deliveries. Any abnormality will be dealt with by a neighbouring maternity hospital. The mother will usually remain in the home until the baby is at least 6 weeks old. If the mother wishes to keep the baby but must work, the baby can be cared for by a foster mother. Adoption of the baby can also be arranged.

Foster Parents

Foster parents are employed by the Social Services Department of the Local Authority and paid by them, but the baby's mother pays according to her means. The foster mother and her home have to be approved. Regular inspection of foster children is undertaken by Health Visitors and Social Workers.

Adoption

A single woman or couple who feel they are unable to keep their baby can apply for the baby to be adopted. This can only be done through a Registered Adoption Society which may be the Social Services Committee of the Local Authority or a religious order.

The baby as a rule will not come under the care of the adoptive parents before 6 weeks of age, in case the legitimate parent or parents change their mind. The baby must remain in the care of the proposed adoptors for at least 3 months before legal adoption procedures can be completed, thus the child will then be at least $4\frac{1}{2}$ months old. Prior to adoption the baby has to be examined medically and a full report submitted to the adoption society. The adoptive parents are also medically examined and full consideration given to their reasons for wishing to adopt a child.

Couples wishing to adopt should usually be between the ages of 25–45; single women and men can adopt under certain conditions, but this is usually discouraged, and normally a male cannot adopt a female child. Prior to legal adoption the case is submitted to a magistrate or County Court. After the court judgement the natural mother has no claim on her child without an appeal.

An adopted child becomes a natural child of the adopting family but is unable to claim hereditary titles.

HEALTH VISITORS

Health visitors may also be midwives but more commonly have obtained the Period 1 Central Midwives Board Certificate or undertaken three months obstetric nurse training. They are employed by Area Health Authorities.

Health visitors supervise clinics held in Personal and Child Health Centres, visit defaulters and take over the care of the mother and child after the patient has been discharged from hospital or after the domiciliary midwife has ceased to visit. It is essential that midwives and health visitors co-operate to ensure continuity of care. Sometimes health visitors and domiciliary midwives attend a general practitioners' surgery to help with well-baby clinics and antenatal clinics respectively. In some areas health visitors pay regular visits to their local maternity hospital. Domiciliary midwives may be called upon to care for mothers and babies who have been delivered in hospital, but sent home within 8 days. Married midwives find this work suitable because as a rule there is no night work.

Maternity hospitals usually employ a *medical social worker* to advise patients how to secure any necessary social help.

FAMILY PLANNING

Midwives should be taught about the various methods available for birth control and ensure that patients know where to apply for advice.

Many obstetric hospitals conduct their own Birth Control (family planning) Clinics usually only for patients with medical abnormalities.

Many couples are happy if a conscientious husband uses a sheath and the wife a spermocidal pessary; sometimes the wife prefers to be fitted with a Dutch Cap. Hormone (pill) tablets are widely used but are contra-indicated if the patient has varicose veins, hypertension, any renal disease or diabetes. An intrauterine coil is an alternative method but can cause damage to a patient with any previous uterine operation, including Caesarean Section.

If the couple have enough children sterilisation should be considered; this can be done on the woman in the early puerperium by a small abdominal incision. Sometimes the husband will consider vasectomy instead.

Family planning advice and treatment is now free. Apart from maternity hospitals, family planning care is done in Area Health Authority clinics and in many general practitioner surgeries. There is also a team of domiciliary family planning nurses who visit patients at home; they often take an interpreter with them if the patient does not speak English. The fertile Asian immigrants benefit from this service.

21 MORTALITY

I MATERNAL MORTALITY

This includes any woman dying as a result of childbirth. The cause may be due to a direct obstetrical complication or to a previous disease aggravated by pregnancy.

Every death is a tragedy. Each case in Britain is investigated thoroughly and there have been seven Ministry of Health and Social Security publications on maternal mortality. The maternal mortality rate is expressed as the number of maternal deaths per 1000 total births (live and still). This rate has fallen dramatically during the last 30 years and is now about 0·15 per 1000. Abortions account for a number of maternal deaths but there are no statistics for the incidence of abortions. Probably about 1 in 20 pregnancies end as an abortion.

All three published reports show that about 50 per cent of the deaths should have been prevented. Sometimes the patient was at fault, failing to obtain medical aid in time, or refusing hospital admission. Sometimes the midwife or doctor failed to detect an abnormality in time and, occasionally, the hospital treatment was faulty.

The relative frequency of causes of maternal deaths keeps changing. According to the last survey *abortion* now heads the list. Deaths due to abortion are usually from sepsis, haemorrhage or injury, and the abortion has generally been illegally performed. This high mortality figure is certainly one reason for the new Abortion Act. Birth Control Councelling is preferable. Usually the women concerned are married with large families.

CAUSES OF MATERNAL DEATHS

(1) Pulmonary Embolism

This is now one of the commonest causes of maternal death. In many of the fatal cases no anticoagulant therapy had been used. Pulmonary embolism is more likely to occur after an operative delivery or complicated labour.

(2) Toxaemia

Toxaemia including accidental haemorrhage. Death can follow eclampsia, haemorrhage, renal cortical necrosis or liver atrophy. Good antenatal care will prevent many of these serious complications, mainly by recognising toxaemia early and admitting patients with toxaemia to hospital for constant observation. Until the exact cause of toxaemia has been determined, the occasional death will occur.

(3) Haemorrhage

This may be associated with placenta praevia or a post partum haemorrhage. Deaths from the former can be prevented if the significance of a 'warning show' is appreciated by patients, midwives and doctors. Patients liable to have a PPH must be delivered in hospital.

Deaths from haemorrhage have been greatly reduced since midwives have been permitted to give oxytoxic drugs after the second stage of labour, and since 'Flying Squads' have become available. Nevertheless, anaemia must be recognised and treated during pregnancy. Routine haemoglobin investigations must be made throughout pregnancy.

(4) Sepsis

Sepsis used to be a common cause of death. Now it is rare; provided suitable preventative measures are taken and infection recognised and treated early with effective antibiotics.

(5) Rupture of the Uterus

Rupture of the uterus usually causes severe haemorrhage and a high mortality. In the past a ruptured uterus usually followed a prolonged labour due to disproportion or a malpresentation, especially shoulder. Nowadays, the rupture is more commonly associated with a previous Caesarean Section scar or after the uterus has been injured by previous curettage. After a Caesarean Section all subsequent deliveries should be in hospital and the patient observed closely for signs of maternal distress.

(6) Anaesthetic Deaths

Anaesthetic deaths can follow inhaled vomitus. The incidence has been reduced by the use of local anaesthesia instead of general anaesthesia for vaginal deliveries. Only specialist anaesthetists should administer a general anaesthetic during labour, and whenever possible the patient should be prevented from having solid food, or glucose drinks during labour.

(7) Associated Diseases

Associated diseases which account for some maternal deaths include:

(a) *Heart disease.* If the heart lesion is recognised early and the patient receives adequate hospital care, a maternal death is rare. The published reports include patients who have died after a home confinement. This is deplorable.

(b) *Pulmonary tuberculosis* used to be associated with a high maternal mortality. This was reduced considerably after the discovery of effective antituberculosis drugs, and when chest X-ray examination in pregnancy became a routine procedure.

II INFANT MORTALITY

Still-births

A still-birth is a baby born after 28 weeks gestation, showing no sign of life, i.e. failing to breathe. Fetal death can occur before or during labour. If the fetus has been dead for over 6 hours when born, the skin shows signs of maceration. A still-birth must be registered by a parent. The still-birth rate is the number of still-births per 1000 total births (live and still).

Neonatal Deaths

A neonatal death is when a baby born alive dies within 28 days of birth. The neonatal death rate is the number of neonatal deaths per 1000 live births. The majority occur within the first 7 days. For this reason and because the aetiology of still-births and early neonatal deaths is frequently identical, the term *perinatal mortality* has been introduced.

Perinatal Deaths

Perinatal deaths include all still-births and deaths of babies before the age of 7 days. The perinatal death rate is the number of perinatal deaths per 1000 total births (live and still).

A national survey of perinatal deaths was undertaken in 1958 and the findings have been published. The perinatal death rate varies from country to country and even in different areas of Great Britain. The national average has now been reduced to about 22. The main causes of death are:

(1) Toxaemia

In severe cases the fetus may die *in utero*. Until the cause of toxaemia is determined, some deaths are inevitable.

(2) Prematurity and Low Birth Weight

A baby born before 37 weeks gestation or with a birth weight below 2500 g has a high mortality. Obstetricians and midwives should endeavour to prevent premature births. The causes of such births include, toxaemia, multiple pregnancy. placenta praevia, a diet deficient in protein, and overwork of the pregnant woman. Occasionally a threatened premature labour can be stopped by giving duvadilan.

Very premature babies may die because of their immature vital organs, and for survival specialised care is essential. Premature and low birth weight babies are liable to die from respiratory disease, and occasionally from intracranial haemorrhage. During labour sedative drugs can be dangerous, as can a reduction of inhaled oxygen. Pressure on the soft premature fetal skull can, in certain cases, be minimised by performing an episiotomy. Ideally, a paediatrician should be present when these babies are born in case the baby is asphyxiated, when mechanical and chemical resuscitation may be required. Nursing thereafter should be in a special baby care unit.

(3) Intracranial Birth Injury

This has been reduced since difficult vaginal deliveries have been replaced by Caesarean Section. Premature babies are liable to injury as are babies born as a breech. For the latter a skilled obstetrician should be present.

(4) Asphyxia

Asphyxia is a risk in any complicated delivery, including Caesarean Section. Modern resuscitation is necessary to prevent some deaths. Prolonged asphyxia may lead to later spasticity or submental development. A postmature placenta may cause asphyxia.

(5) Congenital Malformation

An abnormal chromosome count, infection during the first three months of pregnancy, e.g. rubella, or drugs taken at that time by the pregnant woman, e.g. thalidomide, are known causes. Many abnormalities occur without obvious reason.

Grossly malformed fetuses tend to abort or are incompatible with survival, e.g. anencephaly, renal agenesis. Some, e.g. oesophageal atresia, if recognised early will respond to surgery.

(6) Infection

With modern antibiotics perinatal death from sepsis has been reduced. However, Gram-negative bacilli may cause a fatal infection. Prevention and early treatment is imperative.

Other causes of infant death include haemolytic disease of: he new-born, especially due to rhesus immunisation and maternal diabetes.

INDEX